Natural Cures
"They" Don't Want You
to Know About

Natural Cures
"They" Don't Want You
to Know About

KEVIN TRUDEAU

Alliance Publishing Group, Inc.

This edition published by Alliance Publishing Group, Inc. For information, address Alliance Publishing Group, Inc., 104 W. Chestnut St.
#330, Hinsdale, Illinois 60521-3387.

ISBN 0-9755995-0-X

Library of Congress EPCN application in process.

Library of Congress Control Number: 2004111635

Manufactured in the United States of America

10 9

Contents

Disclaimer

It is unbelievable to me, in this day and age, that the world has come to this. It pains me that I must write a disclaimer at the beginning of this book. Imagine, a person who is supposed to be allowed to express his opinions under the banner of "free speech" must still put a disclaimer as a preface to his words, thoughts and opinions. Heaven forbid someone reads these words and claims to be adversely affected by them, thus ensuring a barrage of lawsuits filed under the guise of protecting the unknowing victims who were stupid enough to read this and believe it! In reality, these lawyers are squashing the rights of people, like myself, from freely expressing their ideas. So with a figurative gun to my head I write these words:

Before you read this book you had better check with your medical doctor, your friends, your politicians, your priest, your rabbi, your psychic and anyone you feel is smarter than you, and see if you can get permission to read what I have to say.

You must know that everything I say in this book is simply my opinion, and that there are many people who violently disagree with my conclusions. If you do anything I recommend without the supervision of a licensed medical doctor, you do so at your own risk. The publisher and the author, the distributors and bookstores, present this information for **educational purposes only***. I am not making an attempt to prescribe any medical treatment, since under the laws of the United States only a licensed medical doctor (an MD) can do so. How sad!*

So this book is only **my** *opinions,* **my** *thoughts and* **my** *conclusions. Again, it is for educational purposes only, and you and only you are responsible if you choose to do anything based on what you read.*

Kevin Trudeau

I Should Be Dead By Now

Great spirits have always encountered violent opposition from mediocre minds.
                                                        —Albert Einstein

I was driving down the Tri-State Highway outside of Chicago, Illinois in my brand new Corvette enjoying a beautiful sunny day. Suddenly I felt an enormous ripping pain in my chest. I could barely breathe; the pain was excruciating. I immediately pulled off to the side of the road. My life virtually flashed before my eyes and I thought, "Oh my god I'm having a heart attack and I'm only twenty-one years old!"

Just as quickly as the pain came, it vanished. I was dizzy, disoriented and in a state of shock and disbelief as to what had just happened. I looked down and noticed my new car phone, an invention that had just come out in the Chicago-land area. I picked up my phone, called my secretary and said "I think I just had a heart attack."

Luckily for me, within a few moments I felt fine. I concluded that if it was a heart attack, it certainly didn't cause any major damage. But something was obviously wrong.

Over the next week I was examined by three of the top heart specialists in America. Through use of the most advanced medical diagnostic devices, it was concluded after days of testing that I had been

1

born with a deformed heart, a severe *mitral valve prolapse* which would cause me major medical problems the rest of my life. There was no cure.

These top medical minds recommended experimental drugs or risky surgery, both of which I was told had little promise. My life expectancy was to be very short. I struggled with coming up with an effective plan of action that could solve my medical dilemma. I was twenty-one years old and had my whole life in front of me. I had to do something!

Months earlier I had attended a lecture where I heard about a Harvard medical doctor named Tang who, during the Korean War, was a MASH surgeon. This MD had decided that standard medical procedures, drugs and surgery were not the best way to cure and prevent diseases. He instead was using a diagnostic device developed in Germany by a Dr. Reinhold Voll called the *Dermatron* machine. Allegedly, in a matter of minutes, it could diagnose medical problems in the body. When the diagnosis was complete, homeopathic remedies were given to correct the imbalances and reverse and cure the disease.

At the time it sounded like hocus pocus. The words homeostasis, holistic healing, homeopathic remedies, acupuncture meridians, energy frequencies, imbalances and the like were used in the lecture, replacing what was, to me, the standard vernacular of germs, bacteria, virus, drugs, surgery and genetics. Skeptical, yet open to new ideas, I flew to Reno, Nevada to meet this great Dr. Tang. What did I have to lose?

Upon my arrival, the doctor asked me why I was there. I looked fit and healthy, and being so young, he was slightly puzzled by my desire for diagnosis. Most of his patients were old and had severe medical problems. Wanting to see if this *Dermatron* machine was legitimate, I simply said, "I feel great. I just want a basic checkup."

Immediately he tested me with his magic machine. Within two minutes he had touched my heart meridian with the probe and the machine registered very low energy. The doctor looked at me, slightly concerned, and said, "Son you have a heart problem." I was shocked at how quickly the diagnosis came. Just as quickly he stated, "Let me find out where it is."

He began to touch other meridian points. When he got to the mitral valve, the machine again registered very little energy. He looked at me and said matter-of-factly, "You have a mitral valve prolapse."

Needless to say, I was quite impressed. The expert medical doctors took days of diagnostic testing to determine that I had a severe mitral valve prolapse. This "energy machine" diagnosed the problem within minutes. I looked at the doctor and said, "Yes I know, and I understand it is incurable." His response startled me. "Yes, in America it's incurable, but there are natural treatments in other countries that can reverse this problem in a matter of weeks. Unfortunately the FDA has not approved these treatments. So yes, in America it is incurable." He then went on to explain a procedure of live cell injections—available in Switzerland or Mexico, but not accessible via legal treatment in the United States—that would correct the problem by actually rebuilding the heart, ensuring that it would never return.

Quite frankly, I couldn't believe my ears. Natural treatments *that work* that are not approved by the FDA? Impossible!

This event happened over twenty years ago. The treatment I received was inexpensive, all-natural, painless, quick, and it worked! And still to this day, that therapy is illegal in America. The most amazing part of this story is, after I received the natural treatment that was forbidden in America, I went back to the medical doctors who originally diagnosed my heart problem and asked to be tested again. My request was met with indignation; I was told that being tested again was a waste of time and money because it was impossible for the medical condition to change in two months. Nevertheless, I demanded a re-administering of all the tests anyway. The doctors humored me, and were stunned when they found I no longer had a mitral valve prolapse.

I was so excited to share with them information about the treatment I had received which had cured my problem. Certainly these doctors would want to know about an all-natural medical treatment that could cure the incurable! Imagine my shock when I was told that the treatment I received could not have cured my disease, but rather I must have been misdiagnosed in the first place and never had the heart deformity to begin with. I could not believe my ears! These medical

doctors would not accept the fact: I had a severe mitral valve prolapse—the pictures confirmed it; and now I do not have a mitral valve
prolapse—the pictures confirm it.

I began to think of all of the people that would come to these
medical doctors and be told the bold face lie that their medical condition was incurable and could only be treated with drugs and
surgery. It sickened me to know that the truth about natural cures
would be hidden from millions of patients. The knowledge that the
established medical community would deny the existence of natural
cures, thus allowing millions of people to suffer and in many cases
die, enraged me.

That event started me on a lifelong mission: searching for natural
remedies that do not include drugs or surgery, and natural treatments
that can prevent and cure illness and disease. It also exposed me to the
organizations, companies and government agencies that do not want
you to know about these cures.

Today I live a full, healthy, dynamic life. I take no drugs and have
had no surgeries. I haven't had a prescription or nonprescription drug
in over twenty years. Additionally, I virtually never get sick. Colds, flus
and all illnesses seem to pass me by. I have had hundreds of blood tests
and other diagnostic tests performed on me every few years, just to
make sure everything is within the normal range. The medical professionals who have examined and reviewed these results are stunned and
amazed at the level of health that I enjoy. Am I lucky? Is it just genetics? Or are there some specific things that a person can do to have a
disease- and illness-free life and enjoy dynamic, vibrant health? Is it
possible for you to go week after week, year after year, and never get
sick? I strongly believe the answer is yes. This book outlines specifically the following things:

- Yes—there are all-natural, nondrug and nonsurgical cures for most
  every illness and disease.

- Yes—there are organizations, government agencies, companies and
  entire industries that are spending billions of dollars trying to hide
  these natural cures from you.

- Yes—*every* single nonprescription and prescription drug has adverse side effects, and should virtually never be taken (with exceptions that I will explain later).

In this book, it's important to note that I am over-simplifying everything. The reason is that I am not writing this book for the medical community, the scientists, researchers or MDs. They are not going to believe or agree with anything I say anyway. I'm writing this book in plain English so that you can understand it.

Let me point out a couple of things. Everything I say in this book is my opinion. Everything stated is what I believe to be true. All my conclusions and statements of fact are, in most cases, opinions.

It's interesting to note that medical science always presents things as fact, when actually what they are really presenting is not fact at all. It's only an *opinion,* based on the information they have at the current time. Throughout history, medical "facts" have been proven not to be true over and over again. Therefore they are not facts at all; they are simply *opinions.* Medical science has stated things to be true and, in most cases, years later those things have been found not to be true. Medical science is almost always wrong, yet they present things as factual, as if they "know" the truth.

The medical industry presents itself as the only source of truth when it comes to health, illness and disease. They use words like *credible scientific evidence, scientifically tested, scientifically proven.* The fact is that what they are really presenting are theories, and these theories constantly change. Here is an example of "medical facts" that have been proven to be wrong:

- Bloodletting was proven to cure most illnesses. Now it is considered totally ineffective.
- Margarine was considered much healthier than butter. Now research suggests that the exact opposite is true.
- Eggs were considered very bad because of high cholesterol. Now research suggests that they are not bad at all, and they are actually healthy for the body.

- Alcohol in all forms was said to be 100 percent unhealthy, and therefore should not be consumed. Then the medical community said that red wine is actually healthy for the heart, but not other forms of alcohol. Now "medical science" says that all alcohol in moderation actually has health benefits.

- Chocolate and oily foods were touted to be a cause of acne. Now research suggests that they do not contribute in any way to acne.

- Homosexuality was once classified as a disease.

- Medical doctors touted that baby formula was much better than breast milk for children. Now the exact opposite is shown to be true.

- Milk was recommended for coating the stomach and alleviating stomach ulcers. Now it is discouraged and has been found to aggravate ulcers.

- Medical science stated that diet had absolutely no effect on disease or illness. Now we are told that diet has a huge effect on the prevention and cause of disease.

- Medical science proved that the removing of tonsils and appendix improved health and should be done to virtually everyone. Now the medical community has reversed that theory.

- Children with asthma were told to stay in enclosed pool areas because the humidity was good for their asthmatic condition. Now research suggests that the chlorine in the air from the pools actually aggravates and makes the asthma worse.

- The most obvious example of all is the fact that there are thousands of drugs that have been approved by the FDA because they were scientifically proven to cure or prevent disease, in addition to having been touted as safe. Then, years later, they have been taken off the market because they had been newly proven to either not cure or prevent those diseases as originally thought, or those drugs were found to have such terribly adverse side effects that they are simply too dangerous for people to use.

The point is, what we are being told by the medical community as "fact" is simply not fact at all. It is the "current theory" and "thought of the day," which historically is often shown to be not true. It saddens me when I see doctors on TV stating things as fact when they should be qualifying their comments with such phrases as *"it appears, based on the current research we have; It seems that; We believe this to be true, however, we also know that as more research and observations are evaluated this may change in the future."* This is not happening. Medical doctors are still looked on as gods. Whatever they say is taken as absolutely true. No one else can say anything about health, illness or disease with the credibility of a medical doctor. That simply is wrong. Medical doctors are only trained to do two things: prescribe drugs, or cut out parts of a person's anatomy (surgery). They are not trained at preventing disease and, most importantly, they have little to no training in or exposure to any treatment other than drugs or surgery.

Another example of medical facts reversed is the diet industry. First, a low calorie diet was said to be the only way to lose weight. Then experts said "It's not the calories, but the amount of fat you consume that will determine your weight." Now the rage of the day is "It's not the calories and it's not the fat, it's the carbohydrates that cause obesity."

The fact is, nobody really knows. Imagine the government's highest medical authority making this statement: "Today we have more information and knowledge about the cure and prevention of disease than ever before in the history of mankind. The advancements that have been made in just the last few years have given us new insights about the treatment and prevention of virtually all illness and disease, making it safe to reach two major conclusions:

1. Even though just ten years ago we thought we knew the proper treatments of illness, we now know just how little we knew back then.

2. With these revolutionary breakthroughs in technology, virtually all illness and disease should be wiped out in America within the next ten years. We are on the verge of being in a place where a person will never be sick. And if you do get sick, your doctor will be able to cure you of your illness in a matter of days. We have virtually reached the pinnacle of medical knowledge."

Sounds exciting, doesn't it? Wow! We have reached the pinnacle of medical knowledge. We know all there is to know about the cure and prevention of disease. Wow! In just ten years, because of medical science, sickness will be eliminated in America. Well, even though it sounds exciting, there is a downside: Imagine that the speech was given in 1902. Interesting, isn't it? In 1902, the people of the day believed they knew all there was to know about the cure and prevention of disease. We look back at them and are in awe at just how little they knew. Now here is the hard part for us to imagine. Twenty years from now, people will look at us and be in awe of how little we know about the cure and prevention of disease. Today we laugh at the thought of bloodletting curing a disease. Well, fifty years from now people will laugh when they look at some of the archaic and horrible treatments that we are using today in an attempt to cure illness.

As you read this book, imagine me prefacing everything I say with *"It seems"* or *"It appears based on current observations and current research…"* I believe this to be true. I know that, of everything I say in this book, as more research and data becomes available, there is an excellent chance that many of these theories and opinions may be altered, modified, improved, or changed completely. Please just note this: *There are virtually no medical facts.* There are only medical opinions. You need to choose the opinion that makes the best sense for you.

How did I come up with my opinions? I have traveled over five million miles to bring you this information. I have been in all fifty U.S. states and traveled to countries all over the world. Over the last twenty years I have talked with thousands of healthcare providers. I have listened to tens of thousands of people who have had serious medical conditions cured by natural therapies, many after drugs and surgery had failed them. I have personally seen with my own eyes, heard with my own ears, and experienced firsthand so much information that I believe I have the unique perspective necessary to come up with my bold conclusions. The biggest acknowledgment I must give is to the tens of thousands of dedicated healthcare professionals around the world who refuse to use drugs and surgery, yet routinely see their patients cured of diseases and living vibrant, healthy lives. These natural healthcare providers see people cured of cancer, diabetes, heart disease, chronic pain, headaches, arthritis, allergies, depression and the list goes on. The question is no longer whether diseases can be prevented or cured faster and more effectively without drugs and surgery. The real question is why is a healthcare provider, who does not use drugs and surgery, being prosecuted as a criminal because he is curing cancer, AIDS or other diseases. Natural therapies work. Natural therapies can work better than drugs or surgery. People who are using natural therapies to cure and prevent disease, and have a higher success rate with no adverse side effects than drug or surgery-type treatments, are being prosecuted for breaking the law. The question is, why are inexpensive, all-natural, safe, effective treatments being suppressed? Let's find out.

C H A P T E R   2

What's Wrong with Healthcare in America

Medical science has absolutely, 100 percent, failed in the curing and prevention of illness, sickness and disease. Consider the following startling bits of data:

- More people get colds and flus than ever before.
- More people get cancer than ever before.
- More people have diabetes than ever before.
- More people have heart disease than ever before.
- More people have multiple sclerosis, lupus, muscular dystrophy, asthma, migraine headaches, joint, neck and back pain than ever before.
- More people have acid reflux, ulcers, and stomach problems than ever before.
- More women have menopause problems than ever before.
- More women have more frequent PMS and more severe PMS than ever before.
- More kids have attention deficit disorder and hyperactivity than ever before.
- More people have chronic fatigue than ever before.
- More people have insomnia than ever before.
- More people have bad skin, acne and dandruff than ever before.

- More people suffer from depression, stress, and anxiety than ever before.
- More men and women suffer from sexual dysfunction and infertility than ever before.
- More people suffer from allergies, arthritis, constipation, fibromyalgia, cold sores, and herpetic breakouts than ever before.
- More men suffer from prostate problems than ever before.
- More women suffer from yeast infections than ever before.

Yet surprisingly enough...

- There are more people going to visit doctors than ever before.
- There are more people getting diagnostic testing, such as blood tests and x-rays, than ever before.
- More people are taking nonprescription and prescription drugs than ever before
- Not only are more people taking drugs, but each person is taking more drugs than ever before.
- There are more surgeries performed than ever before.

What does this tell us? It tells us that standard medical science is failing. More people are getting medical treatment, taking more drugs, having more diagnostic testing and having more surgeries than ever before in history. Yet more people are getting sick than ever before in history. Medical science is failing! According to *Fortune* magazine we are losing the war on cancer. The percentage of Americans dying of cancer today is the same as it was in 1970 and even 1950! Over $200 billion has been spent since 1971 trying to prevent and cure cancer. Yet today you have a higher chance of getting cancer than ever before in history, and you have the same chance of dying as you did in 1950. I would call that a miserable failure. Americans spend over $2 trillion a year on healthcare, yet the American infant mortality rate is higher than twenty other developed countries. People in thirty other countries live longer than Americans, yet, Americans consume over half of all the drugs manufactured in the world. There are over 200,000 nonprescription drugs on the market; there are over 30,000 prescription medications. Doctors write over three billion prescriptions each year. The average American has over thirty different prescription and non-prescription drugs in their medicine cabinet. The bottom line: The only winners in the cure and prevention of disease are the drug companies and the healthcare companies themselves. The drug companies' profits are at an all-time high. Medical science has failed unequivocally in the prevention and curing of virtually every illness.

As an example, let's look at the "Diet Industry":

• More people are on diets than ever before.
• More people take more diet products than ever before.
• More people exercise than ever before.
• Yet more people are fat than ever before. Over 68 percent of the people living in America are overweight. It's been increasing virtually every single year. Not only are more people fatter than ever before, more people are dangerously obese!

Who are the winners in the war on obesity? The corporations that sell diet food, diet pills, and other weight loss aids are making more money than ever before.

An ideal scenario would be never having to take a single drug and never getting sick. An ideal scenario would be waking up in the morning full of energy and vitality, content and feeling absolutely great. You go throughout your day with energy, a bounce in your step, a smile on your face. You don't feel stressed, anxious, or depressed; you don't feel tired, you have no headaches or pain in your body; you are not overweight and you don't get colds or flus or sickness. You don't get diseases, you have no pain, you're not ravenous with your appetite, you eat what you want and you are never that hungry. You don't deprive yourself of the foods you enjoy. You go to sleep at night and you sleep soundly and peacefully and get a wonderful whole night's rest. Your sexual desires are healthy and strong, and you are capable of both giving and receiving sexual pleasure. Your skin, your hair and your nails look healthy and radiant. You have strength and tone in your muscles. Your body is fluid, graceful and flexible. You are firm, strong, vibrant, and feel great!

This is the description of a healthy person. A healthy person never has to take a drug. A healthy person never has to have surgeries. A healthy person has no cancer, diabetes or heart disease. A healthy person lives without illness, sickness or disease. Most people have no idea how good their body is designed to feel. We have been brainwashed into believing that it is natural for a human being to get colds and flus, have aches and pains, and have major medical problems like cancer, diabetes and heart disease. We are also brainwashed into believing that it's "natural" to take drugs. We are programmed to believe that it is normal and natural to take drugs and that we "need" drugs in order to be healthy. Consider this—animals in the wild, such as chimpanzees, do not get sick! They do not get diabetes, cancer, heart disease, asthma, heart burn, arthritis, etc. Animals in the wild also do not take drugs. Animals in the wild don't go to the health club to work out. Yet without drugs, medical visits, surgeries or formalized exercise routines, animals in the wild have virtually no disease or illness and live three to five times longer than humans. The point is, you do not have to get sick. Being sick is not "normal," it is abnormal. Most people think they are healthy, but they really have no idea just how good they could feel.

Is there a place for surgery and drugs? The answer is absolutely yes! Medical science has done a very good job at addressing symptoms. However, the treatment of a symptom has two flaws. First, the treatment itself usually causes more problems which will have to be treated later. Secondly, the cause of the symptom is usually never addressed. When you do not address the cause, you are allowing for problems later on. With this said, if you are in an emergency situation such as that caused by a sudden accident of some sort, drugs and surgery can save your life. However, drugs and surgery have failed at preventing illness and they do not address the cause of illness. Nevertheless, they do work well in emergency crisis situations. The bottom line is, if you fall off a ladder and puncture a kidney, you want to be rushed to the closest emergency room and have a trained medical doctor use drugs and surgery to save your life. But if you want to stay healthy and never have disease, drugs and surgery are not the answer. I will explain this in more detail in a later chapter.

So if trillions of dollars in scientific research has failed in producing ways to prevent and cure illness and disease, and all-natural inexpensive prevention methods and cures do exist, why aren't we hearing about them? The answer may surprise you.

It's All About the Money

Profit is not a four letter word, but rape is against the law.
—**Author Unknown**

My contention is that there are all-natural cures for virtually every disease and ailment. These cures are being suppressed and hidden from you by the pharmaceutical industry, the Food and Drug Administration and the Federal Trade Commission, as well as other groups. The question that arises most often when I make these statements is "What is the motive for such a thing to occur?" The answer is simple: money and power. Most people have no idea just how powerful a motivating force money and power can be. Money does indeed make the world go round. The love of money, which is the definition of greed, is in fact the root of all evil. Think about some obvious facts. Ninety percent of all people in prison today are there because of a money related crime. Interesting isn't it? Money is such a powerful force people will risk going to jail for it. Seventy-five percent of all murders are committed for money. People's insatiable desire to have money actually drives them to kill another human being!

All publicly traded corporations have a legal responsibility to increase profits, it's the law! Think about it: With rare exception, every single

17

business has one objective—to make more profits. The only way companies make more profits is by producing their product at the lowest possible cost, selling it at the highest possible price, and selling as much as they can. Every decision a company makes is to increase profits.

Companies, however, are run by people. People have two motivations—first, to make more money for themselves personally; and secondly, to increase their power, prestige or influence. Therefore, the individuals who run companies will always make decisions based on what can personally enrich themselves. Very few individuals are concerned about the good of mankind, the environment or achieving some spiritual nirvana. To varying degrees, decisions are based on the answer to the question "What's in it for me?"

In business, is everything always about the money? Yes. Throughout the history of big business, *planned obsolescence* has been standard operating procedure. This is when a product is manufactured in such a way so that it will wear out or need to be replaced. The product could have been made to last a very long time; but in order for the company to ensure future profits, it knowingly manufactured an item that was inherently flawed. Thus it planned for the product's obsolescence, all in the name of profit.

In today's business environment, companies only do things that either increase sales, decrease the cost of the product, or guarantee a higher price for the product. A simplified example of this is the restaurants concession in airports. The restaurant has a monopoly, there is no competition. Since the restaurant knows it is not relying on repeat business, it does not have to give good quality food, good service, or a fair price. Have you ever gotten a great meal with great service at a great price at an airport restaurant? I sure haven't. Why? Because they don't have to. Giving good service and a good product at a fair price will not increase profit at an airport restaurant because they are not relying on repeat customers. Another example is outsourcing. Why are hundreds of companies laying off millions of American workers, and outsourcing this work to people in other countries? Because it's cheaper! Remember, the corporate officers and directors of publicly traded companies have a legal responsibility to increase profits. If they don't they will lose their jobs.

Big business will always make decisions based on profit, not what is good for the employees, what is good for the customer, what is good for the environment, what is good for society, or what is good for mankind.

Let's look at the drug industry. Let's say you sell insulin to diabetics. Would you be happy if someone discovered an herb that when taken cured a person's diabetes so that they never needed insulin again? Of course not. You would be out of business. As an interesting note, there is such a cure for diabetes. The person who discovered it was offered over $30 million by a major pharmaceutical company **not to market it!** It's all about the money.

Healthcare, defined as the cure, prevention, and diagnosis of disease, is the most profitable industry in the world. As long as people are sick, billions and billions of dollars in profit are made every year. Think about it. There are enormous amounts of money to be made as long as people stay sick. A healthy person, on the other hand, doesn't spend any money on the healthcare industry. A healthy person does not need to buy drugs, does not get medical treatment, and is a liability to the corporations involved in healthcare. If every person was healthy and disease free, the drug companies and virtually the entire healthcare industry would be out of business. To the drug companies and virtually all the corporations involved in healthcare, you are nothing more than a customer. As long as you are sick you are potentially a good customer. There is no financial incentive for the healthcare industry in having people live disease free. There is no financial incentive to prevent or cure disease. Rather, the entire healthcare industry is driven by one overshadowing motive: to make money! The entire healthcare industry is run by individual people in the form of officers and directors of the publicly traded corporations that make up the industry. These people are, with rare exception, some of the most ruthless, wealthiest, and greediest people on the planet. Is this true? Let's examine a fictitious—or maybe not so fictitious—scenario.

• • •

Imagine there is a scientist working in a lab somewhere. He makes a breakthrough discovery: A small plant is found in the Amazon that, when made into a tea and consumed, eliminates all cancer in the body within one week. Imagine this researcher proclaiming that he has given this tea to one thousand cancer patients, and that every single one of them, within one week and without having undergone surgery, was found to have absolutely no cancer in their body. Eureka! A cure for cancer! A simple, inexpensive, all-natural cure with no side effects. Just a simple plant that you make into a tea and drink. It has absolutely no side effects at all. It's pure, all-natural, and costs just pennies.

Imagine this scientist announcing his discovery to the world. Certainly he would win a Nobel Prize. Certainly the world medical community would be rejoicing. No more cancer! Every cancer patient could drink this tea and in one week be free of all their cancer. Every person who lives with the fear of getting cancer could now know that they could simply drink a few cups of this tea, which costs them only a few pennies, and they could avoid ever getting cancer. My, my, the world would be a better place.

Unfortunately, you'll never hear this story. Not because the story is not true, but because if this simple herbal tea which cures all cancer was allowed to be sold, there would be no need for the American Cancer Society. There would be no need for any of the drug companies that are manufacturing and selling cancer drugs. There would be no need for any additional cancer research funding. Cancer clinics around the world would close, hundreds of thousands of people would be put out of work, entire industries would shut down overnight and billions and billions and billions of dollars in profit would no longer be funneling in to the kingpins who control the cancer industry.

So when this person makes this discovery, what happens? In some cases these people simply vanished. In other cases these people were given hundreds of millions of dollars for their research. In still other cases the federal government raided these researchers' offices, confiscated the data and jailed the researchers for practicing medicine without a license. Is this fantasy or is this the truth? Well the healthcare industry has a dirty little secret, and I am blowing the whistle on it.

The conversations I've heard, the meetings I have attended, the papers that I've read and the inside information that I have received about the healthcare fraud going on in this world has made me mad as hell—and I'm not going to take it any more. I've been dubbed "The

Whistleblower" because I am blowing the whistle on the most profitable industry in the world: healthcare. I'm exposing the lies, the frauds, and the scams. I'm letting the cat out of the bag. Like other industries, once the truth is made known, things begin to change.

Is it true that the healthcare industry is holding back natural, inexpensive cures for disease and illness? Could it be true that the only motivation in healthcare is profits? Let's just look at recent history:

We've all heard the stories of the inventors who had carburetors that would make automobiles run a thousand miles to a gallon of gasoline. We've heard that the automobile industry paid off those inventors with millions of dollars to secure the patents, and then buried those patents and never used that technology. Why? Because it would cost the automotive industry billions of dollars in profits.

We all know the story of how the big three automobile manufacturers purchased the Redline Train System in California, only to dismantle it to make sure that more automobiles were sold. Most people don't know that a lawsuit was filed regarding this obvious antitrust issue and the "big three" were found guilty! Corruption runs deep, however, as evidenced by the judge awarding the plaintiffs one dollar in damages. Many of you remember the movie *Tucker,* about the gentleman who invented the revolutionary automobile only to have the automotive industry bankrupt him because he threatened their profits.

Most recently, many of you have seen the movie *The Insider* or read the book about how for years the tobacco industry lied about their knowledge that the ingredients in cigarettes were highly addictive. Finally, an insider blew the whistle and told the truth. He exposed, finally, what we all assumed was true, that the research was conclusive, cigarettes are addictive, and that the manufacturers of cigarettes knew this for years and years and years, but lied before Congress and said that they "have no knowledge" or "credible scientific evidence" that cigarettes are addictive. It was a flat-out lie. Why did they lie? Money. It's all about the money!

I happen to be a capitalist and an entrepreneur, and throughout my life I have been motivated to make money. Money itself is not bad. We have heard the phrase "The love of money is the root of all evil." The more multimillionaires I talk to, the more billionaires I talk to, the more Wall Street insiders I talk to, the more CEOs of major corporations I talk to, the more big business corporate directors I talk to, the more I believe that the love of money is indeed the root of all evil. I can tell you from firsthand experience that the majority of officers and directors of major publicly traded corporations are greedy beyond belief. Making money becomes an addiction. Making more money becomes the all-consuming compulsive motivator of these people. Making money becomes the most important thing in these people's lives. Making money and doing whatever it takes to make more money becomes the chief motivation in virtually all their decisions and actions. If making more money means lying, stealing, defrauding, falsifying or harming other people, it's okay. If making more money means breaking the laws, destroying the environment or seeing other people suffer, it's okay. Don't believe me? Let me point out a few examples:

Did you know there are thousands and thousands of millionaires, multimillionaires, and billionaires in prisons all around the world? Why are they in prison? Because even with their millions, they had such greed that they were willing to break the law to make more money. You may think these people are the exceptions. Consider this: For every drug dealer that was caught and is in prison, there are probably one thousand drug dealers on the streets that were not caught! I can tell you firsthand that for every millionaire or corporate officer or director that is in prison for breaking the law out of greed, there are hundreds if not thousands of officers, directors and wealthy stock holders who are defrauding the public motivated by personal greed. Do you know what the number one motive of murder is? Money! That's right, money. Money and greed are such strong motivators that it is the number one reason a person will kill another human being. It most definitely is true: Greed, defined as the love of money, is indeed the root of all evil.

We see it on TV with Enron and WorldCom and Martha Stewart. Individuals who have tens of millions of dollars in their bank accounts and are so greedy they want more. They will lie and defraud, cheat and effectively steal money from shareholders and employees for their own personal gain. Their ethics have been thrown out the window. They've sold their soul to the devil. It's all about the money. Just watch reality TV! Do you know that the producers of most reality TV shows are hoping that the real people on these shows have their lives ruined on national television? The producers make money with great ratings. If a person is physically hurt or has an emotionally traumatizing event happen, the ratings soar and the producers make more money. The more "bad" that happens to the individual the more money is made. It's like feeding Christians to the lions. Why are people so happy when another person's life has been destroyed on national TV? Because when you are so interested in money. Even voyeuristically, you stop caring about other people's lives.

I've been in the corporate boardrooms. I've listened to these people talk. I've heard first hand, so I know that what I am saying is true; and most importantly, I have been there myself. Greed motivated me to break the rules, and I spent two years in federal prison because of it. Believe me, I know first hand what I am talking about. Why haven't you heard this before? Well, for decades what went on in the mafia was a secret. No one even admitted that La Cosa Nostra existed. Finally, one person, Joe Velacci, came forward and blew the whistle on the inner workings of organized crime. Since that time, dozens of former Mafiosi have come forward to share the secrets that went on behind closed doors. In a similar fashion, the inner workings of the tobacco industry have been shrouded in secrecy. Finally, a man with a conscience came forward at the risk of his own life to blow the whistle on the greed, lies and deceit that was directly responsible for the deaths of hundreds of thousands of people. Think about it. Where are weapons of mass destruction? They are in every package of cigarettes! Today, I am one of the first to come forward from the inside and tell you the truth about the people who run "big pharma." You may be under the illusion that drug companies have officers and directors whose sole passion in life is to prevent and cure disease for the benefit of mankind. But I am pulling back the curtain and exposing the great Oz for the fraud that he really is. You may hear the cry "pay no attention to the man behind the curtain," but do not be deceived. The officers and directors of the big corporations that make up the healthcare industry are not benevolent, wonderful people with compassion and a desire to rid the world of illness. When the curtain is pulled back and the true identities are revealed, we see outrageously wealthy people whose greed, insatiable desire to make more money, and contempt for humanity is startling and mind-blowing. If you'd had the chance to shake these people's hands and look into their eyes, you would no longer feel safe.

Just remember that healthcare is the most profitable industry in the world and as long as people are sick, people are making billions of dollars in profits.

The bottom line is this: The healthcare industry has no incentive for curing disease. If the healthcare industry cured disease they would all be out of business. Their focus, as unbelievable as it sounds, is to ensure more people get sick and more people need medical treatment. That ensures profits. It's all about the money! Hospitals, drug companies and the entire healthcare industry should really be called the "sick care" industry. This money machine does not make their profits by keeping people healthy, but rather finding a sick person and then selling them their outrageously expensive drugs, surgical procedures, and other medical procedures. And they make over $1.3 trillion annually doing it. Folks, I've been in the board rooms. I've listened to these people. I've heard CEOs of major pharmaceutical companies say things such as this: "I don't care how much liver damage this drug causes, get it approved by the FDA. Pay whoever you have to pay, get the lobbyists that you have to get, but just get this drug approved. Do it, and our stock price goes up three-fold. We sell our stock and move on. And five years from now, when they find out about the liver damage, they'll take the drug off the market. But who cares, we'll have our money. Just do it." That is why I am mad as hell, and I am not going to take it anymore.

Is it always just about the money? Are natural remedies and cures being suppressed and hidden from us just because greedy people and corporations want to make more money? Is it true that money makes the world go 'round? Yes! You must understand the number one motivator in the world is making money. We read about it every day. So let's look at who's involved…

Who Are "They"?

The thing that bugs me is that the people think the FDA is protecting them. It isn't. What the FDA is doing and what the public thinks it's doing are as different as night and day. —**Herbert Lay, M.D., former FDA Commissioner**

Drugs and surgery are being promoted as the only answer to the prevention and cure of illness and disease. Natural cures are being suppressed and hidden from the public. So who is involved in this "great lie"? Let me expose the culprits:

- **The Pharmaceutical Companies**—These include not only the companies that sell drugs, but also the companies that research and develop drugs. It also includes all of the suppliers in the healthcare industry of such things as syringes, gauze, medical tape, tubing, plastic bottles, tongue depressors, etc. There are over 10,000 individual pharmaceutical pieces of equipment that are used up and have to be re-supplied on an ongoing basis. The profits are astronomical. The money this group of companies makes is mind boggling.

- **The Food Companies**—You may ask: how do food companies get involved in healthcare? Well there is a huge correlation between food and healthcare. I'll explain this in detail in a later chapter. Keep in mind many food companies are directly or indirectly involved in the pharmaceutical industry through corporate ownership, affiliated business transactions, or by the officers and directors personally owning stock in the pharmaceutical companies. Food companies include the companies that actually manufacture and sell food directly to us, but also includes fast food restaurants and the suppliers of the food industry, the actual growers of the food.

- **The Trade Associations**—The number of associations involved in the healthcare industry is enormous. Keep in mind, these associations are not in place to eliminate disease or keep people healthy. When you read their charters you find that they are there to *promote* the disease, in an effort to get additional funding and protect its members, which are the drug companies and doctors! These associations include:

Alzheimer's Association

American Academy of Allergy, Asthma & Immunology

American Academy of Child and Adolescent Psychiatry

American Academy of Facial Plastic and Reconstructive Surgery

American Academy of Family Physicians

American Academy of Neurology

American Academy of Ophthalmology

American Academy of Orthopedic Surgeons

American Academy of Otolaryngology

American Academy of Otolaryngic Allergy

American Academy of Pediatrics

American Academy of Physical Medicine and Rehabilitation

American Association of Clinical Endocrinologists

American Association of Gynecological Laparoscopists

American Association for Geriatric Psychiatry

American Association of Immunologists

American Association of Neurological Surgeons

American Association for Respiratory Care

American Association for the Study of Liver Diseases

American Board of Medical Specialties

American Board of Ophthalmology

American Board of Psychiatry and Neurology, Inc.

American Cancer Society

American College of Allergy, Asthma and Immunology

American College of Cardiology

American College of Chest Physicians

American College of Gastroenterology

American College of Obstetricians and Gynecologists

American College of Physicians

American College of Rheumatology

American College of Surgeons

American Congress of Rehabilitation Medicine

American Diabetes Association

American Gastroenterological Association

American Geriatrics Society

American Health Information Management Association

American Heart Association

American Liver Foundation

American Lung Association

American Medical Association

American Medical Women's Association

American Neurological Association

American Neurotology Society

American Orthopedic Society for Sports Medicine

American Otological Society

American Osteopathic Association

American Pharmaceutical Association

American Prostate Society

American Psychiatric Association

American Red Cross

American Rhinologic Society

American Society of Clinical Oncology

American Society for Gastrointestinal Endoscopy

American Society for Head and Neck Surgery

American Society of Pediatric Otolaryngology

American Society for Reproductive Medicine

American Urological Association

Association of Telehealth Service Providers

Catholic Health Association of the United States

The Endocrine Society

Gerontological Society of America

Leukemia & Lymphoma Society of America

National Alliance for the Mentally Ill

National Association of Psychiatric Health Systems

National Board for Respiratory Care

National Stroke Association

Society of Gynecologic Oncologists

Vestibular Disorders Association (VEDA)

This list is just the tip of the iceberg. These associations are incredibly powerful. Remember, these associations are not organizations with a goal of curing and preventing disease, or protecting the consumer. These associations do not represent you, they represent their members: the companies, the corporations, and the people that are making the money. Associations such as the American Medical Association have no interest in what benefits the consumer. They only have an interest in what benefits their members. And the people that run these associations have an interest in keeping their high paying cushy jobs.

• **Charities and Foundations**—These organizations sound great, but have you met the people who run them? The officers and directors of most charities and foundations have huge salaries and enormous expense accounts. They fly first-class and sometimes on private jets; they stay in the most expensive hotels and eat in the finest restaurants—all with your donations. Some foundations and charities have been found to spend over 40 percent of all of their donations on "administration costs." Think about it. If a foundation used the money it received to cure a disease, there would be no need for the foundation and the fat cats would lose their prestigious jobs and all the perks that go along with them. Yes, it's always about the money. But consider the second most powerful motivator for people is the combination of power and prestige. Think about that when you ask yourself: "Why are natural cures being hidden from us?" Consider this: The Jerry Lewis Telethon has raised over $1 billion for muscular dystrophy, yet more people have muscular dystrophy today than ever before.

- **Lobbyists**—This is the hidden, secret group of people in Washington that most of you have no idea even exists. These people on average make between $300,000 to $400,000 a year, plus hundreds of thousands more in perks. Their job is simply to walk up to a congressman or senator and try to persuade them to a certain line of thinking, or to pass a certain piece of legislation, or vote a certain way. Now how do they do that? Well, the lobbyist can't walk up to a member of Congress and say "Please vote a certain way on this bill and I will give you $200,000." That would be called a bribe. But what the lobbyist can do is say, "Do you have a son or a daughter, Mr. Congressman? You do? Fantastic! You know, I know your son or daughter has absolutely no experience whatsoever, but we would like to give your son or daughter a job for $200,000 a year. And the best part is they don't even have to show up for work. Oh, by the way Mr. Congressman, can you please vote a certain way on this particular piece of legislation which helps who I represent?" Lobbyists also bribe members of Congress, although Congress has passed laws that make them legally not a bribe, by doing other things. Lobbyists may make huge donations to a congressman's favorite charity or school, or hire companies that the congressman is affiliated with in some way. Folks, that's what is happening in Washington. Lobbyists absolutely bribe and payoff congressmen. But according to the law it is not called a bribe or payoff, it is technically legal. And who makes the law? The Congressmen. Hmm, pretty interesting isn't it? They make a law to make sure that what they do is legal. Can you begin to see why I'm mad a hell and I'm not going to take it anymore?

• **Government Agencies**—Primarily the Food and Drug Administration and the Federal Trade Commission. Isn't it surprising that it's the Food AND Drug Administration? (Why not two separate agencies?) This organization is one of the most powerful organizations in the country. They use Gestapo-like tactics to put natural cures out of business. They act as judge, jury and executioner. They raid companies unannounced to seize products such as bread, herbal remedies, vitamins and minerals, computers, files, research data, and equipment. They conduct these raids with armed agents with guns drawn. They seize harmless products, papers, documents, and computers, like the Gestapo did in Nazi Germany, without provocation, with no customer or consumer complaints, and without warning.

There have been several outstanding books and articles written about how the FDA operates. But in the end, the FDA is the agency that approves drugs. And when a company gets a drug approved, it's like putting billions of dollars in profits in the bank. So companies will do *anything* to get the FDA to approve drugs. It's interesting to note that of the last twenty FDA commissioners, twelve of them went to work directly for the drug industry upon leaving the FDA and were paid millions of dollars. Let's be honest, that's a payoff. It should be illegal; it's a conflict of interest, and it's wrong. More on the FDA in a later chapter.

Ok, now let's go though each of these organizations and let me show you that it is all about the money:

• **The Pharmaceutical Industry**. Virtually every pharmaceutical company is a publicly traded company, which means that the officers and directors have a legal responsibility to increase shareholder value. That means that the officers and directors of virtually every pharmaceutical company have a legal responsibility to increase profits. The only way they can increase profits is to sell more of what they sell and produce those products at a lower cost. Drug companies, therefore, have one goal, and that is to sell more drugs and produce those drugs at the cheapest possible cost. Think about that. A drug company's objective is not to cure disease. A drug company's goal is to sell more drugs. You are their customer. They want you to use more drugs every single year. They want to produce those drugs at the lowest possible cost and they want to do whatever they can to make sure that they can sell those drugs at the highest possible price. That's why there is a huge debate about people buying pharmaceutical drugs from other countries. The FDA makes up this silly excuse that a country like Canada doesn't produce drugs under the same safety guidelines as America. How arrogant!

The fact is that American pharmaceutical companies want a monopoly. They do not want anybody competing with their sales; therefore they have managed to coax the federal government into forbidding any American to purchase a pharmaceutical drug outside of America. They are in effect stopping free trade and stopping competition, which would result in lower prices. Why is the FDA doing that? As I mentioned to you before, the drug industry gives millions of dollars to the commissioners when they leave the FDA. It's a payoff!

Remember: Drug companies do not want people to get well. A drug company's goal is not to cure disease. If everyone in the world was healthy, the drug companies would be out of business. A drug company only wants to sell you more drugs. So here is how the cycle works:

The drug industry gives billions of dollars to medical schools. Why? So that their drugs can be put in the textbooks and doctors are taught to prescribe certain pharmaceutical drugs, thus guaranteeing sales of those drugs by the pharmaceutical company. Remember, in medical school doctors are taught two things: to prescribe drugs and to cut out parts of a person's anatomy, which is surgery.

When a doctor comes out of medical school, most people don't know that the pharmaceutical industry then pays that doctor to prescribe certain drugs. Often, this is done through "incentives." For example, if a doctor prescribes ten patients a certain drug, he is given thousands of dollars in cash from the pharmaceutical company. Drug companies routinely give doctors all expense paid trips to "medical conferences" around the world. These medical conferences are really sales presentations by the drug companies, teaching the doctor about drugs and how to prescribe them, and giving financial incentives to prescribe those drugs. They are disguised as medical conferences. They are not. The experts at these medical conferences are compensated by the drug industry.

So doctors are trained in medical school to prescribe drugs, and are given incentives and additional training throughout their medical career directly by the drug industry to prescribe more drugs.

- **Research**. In order for a drug company to get a drug patented and approved by the FDA, it costs approximately $800 million in research and testing. Where does that $800 million go? Well, let's just follow the money trail. Remember, it's always just about the money!

The companies that are approved by the FDA to do certain research, interestingly enough, are publicly traded companies. Guess who owns the stock in these publicly traded companies? Would it surprise you to know that politicians and members of the FDA own stock in those companies? It wouldn't surprise me! Would it also surprise you that the people that work for those research companies are friends and relatives of politicians and members of the FDA? It wouldn't surprise me!

Once a drug is approved and the pharmaceutical company has the patent, it becomes the only company that can sell that drug. Getting a patented drug is an automatic billion dollars in the bank! This is why you will never see a pharmaceutical company promoting a natural cure. Natural cures can not be patented! You can only make profits if you have a patented drug. There are no large profits in selling a natural cure that can not be patented. When you have a patented product you are the only company that can sell it. You have no competition. You can sell it for an outrageously high price, and the profits are guaranteed. If you are selling a non-patented natural product, a hundred other companies could also sell the same product. You have no monopoly. Because of the competition, the prices will come down and the profits become incredibly small. That is why the drug industry will only promote patented drugs, because that's where the profits are.

So how do the drug companies get you to buy their drugs? Years ago, the drug companies had to basically make sure that you were sick and had a problem that the drug addressed. Secondly, they had to make sure that the doctors prescribed their particular drug. That still goes on. The pharmaceutical companies give huge cash incentives and information to the doctors about the drugs they make to ensure that the doctors, who are in fact legal drug pushers, get their drugs to you via prescription.

Remember, the pharmaceutical companies have ensured that you are sick. How do they do that? This is going to blow your mind, but it's true. One of the major reasons why there is so much sickness and disease is because of the poisons you are putting in your body. The number one poison you put in your body consists of prescription and nonprescription drugs! That's right. The prescription and nonprescription drugs you are taking to eliminate your symptoms are, in fact, one of the major reasons that you get sick.

The pharmaceutical companies know that all drugs have side effects. This is the dirty little secret that the pharmaceutical companies don't want you to know. Just as the tobacco industry knew that smoking cigarettes were addictive and could cause lung cancer, yet lied for decades about this fact, the pharmaceutical industry today knows that all drugs have negative side effects and can cause further illness in the body! The pharmaceutical industry knows that the drugs people are taking are actually causing or contributing to the increases in cancer, heart disease, diabetes and dozens of other diseases. Why is the drug industry keeping this information a secret? Mainly because it's profitable. It is just like the tobacco industry. Look at the cycle: You start taking a drug to handle a certain symptom that you have. A few months later you develop another medical condition. This new medical condition, unknown to you, was actually caused by the first drug you were taking! You now start taking another drug for this new medical condition. The drug seems to work. Your condition gets better. A few months later you develop a new series of medical problems. Unknown to you was the fact that these new medical problems were actually caused by the last drug you were taking. You are given more drugs for this newest medical condition. Can you see how profitable this is for the drug industry? The drug companies are doing this on purpose.

They're making drugs that address one set of symptoms. But they know that if you use these drugs, over a period of time, they can cause a second set of medical problems. The drug companies will then produce a drug to solve those new medical problems caused by taking their first drug. This guarantees additional drug sales and profits for the drug companies.

How is this happening? Keep in mind virtually all drug research is funded by the pharmaceutical industry. In virtually every study, drugs are found to be safe and effective. However, history has proved that this is not true. Think of all of the drugs that were proven to be totally safe and effective and were approved by the FDA. Then, years later these same drugs were proven to be incredibly dangerous and to cause all types of severe medical conditions, including death. These "safe and effective" drugs were found to kill so many people that the FDA finally had to take them off the market. Interestingly enough, they were only taken off the market after the drug companies made millions of dollars in profits.

- **Advertising**. The drug industry is doing something today that it has never done before in history: **advertising its drugs directly to the consumer**. This is absolutely unbelievable! Right now close to two-thirds of all advertising in America is for drugs. It's estimated that well in excess of $10 billion a year is spent on advertising by the pharmaceutical industry. They are advertising drugs directly to you and me, the consumer. In many cases, these drug ads don't even tell you what the drug is for. They just have some celebrity, that they pay huge amounts of money to, telling you about how their life is so much better because they take this particular drug. The ads show all these beautiful happy people and give you the impression that they are all taking this wonderful drug and that their lives are so much better.

What you don't know is that virtually every single person you see in these ads has been meticulously selected by some of the top advertising minds in the world to evoke a certain emotion in you. They are paid actors; most do not use the drug they are promoting. When you see people dressed as doctors, policemen, judges, etc., you are being deceived. Even when known figures and famous actors publicly endorse a drug or foundation (usually funded by pharmaceutical companies), obstensibly because they or a close friend or relative has suffered with a particular disease, they are being paid enormous sums to do so. They are actors. These ads are not truthful. Millions of dollars are spent using technology pioneered by the CIA and KGB to produce advertising that will motivate you to not only want their drug, but feel you *need* their drug. The ads produced by the pharmaceutical industry are the most sophisticated, well though out, brainwashing and manipulating campaigns ever launched on the American public. This advertising is trying to brainwash us into thinking that our life will be better in every way as long as we continue to take more and more drugs. This is absolutely outrageous! Doesn't it drive you crazy when you see all of these drug ads in newspapers, magazines, and television?

The amount of drug advertising is at an all-time high and continues to increase. When you listen to these ads, doesn't it make you smile or laugh when they start rattling off all the side effects of the drugs? However, the marketing techniques are so sophisticated that the drug ads are incredibly effective.

Drug companies get us to use drugs through the use of the media. This is one of the scariest things I want to talk about. The Food and Drug Administration, the Federal Trade Commission and the pharmaceutical industry have an unholy alliance. The regulating government body should be governing and regulating and protecting consumers from the drug companies' incestuous desire to make more profits. The problem is that they work together to increase profits and power.

A law was passed in Congress with virtually no debate at all which increased the FDA's dependence on large drug companies for its funding. You are reading this right. The FDA gets funding directly from the drug industry. It is a law that was passed in 1992 that was intended to speed up approval for new AIDS medications. But what it actually did was get the drug companies to pay for the FDA's new employees and additional funding requirements. According to an article in the *Washington Post,* the program was developed between the pharmaceutical industry and the FDA in secret meetings. It was not debated in Congress, there was no vote. It was a secret, private negotiation between the drug industry and the FDA and went directly to the General Accounting Office for review. According to the *Washington Post,* over 500 new employees to be sent to the FDA centers that actually review new proposed drugs would be paid for by the pharmaceutical and biotechnology companies themselves. There are over 1500 people that work for the FDA who are paid by the funding of the drug industry. That means over 55 percent of the FDA's staff directly involved in the reviewing of new drug applications is in effect on the payroll of the drug industry. That's over $1.2 billion that the FDA is getting directly from the drug industry.

Just to point out how crooked these people are, over the last ten years the FDA has approved over nine specific drugs that have been proven to have deadly side effects. *The Journal of the American Medical Association* estimates that over 125,000 Americans die each year from side effects of FDA approved drugs.

So how do the FDA, FTC, and the drug industry work together promoting drugs and surgery and suppressing natural cures? Criminologist Elaine Feuer did a thorough investigation on the FDA, and found that the FDA invests the majority of its time protecting the profits of the pharmaceutical industry. The FDA suppresses the truth about natural cures and focuses on shutting down companies that sell natural remedies for common diseases. Her book, *Innocent Casualties, the FDA's War Against Humanity,* documents how the FDA specifically goes after companies that offer natural cures for diseases that make the most money for the pharmaceutical industry. Since cancer, AIDS, heart disease and diabetes are so profitable for the drug companies, anyone promoting a natural cure for theses illnesses will be attacked by the FDA. The drug industry, the FTC, and the FDA produce press releases, news if you will, on new super wonder-drugs. At the same time they spread negative news on natural alternatives. The industry spends enormous amounts of money with public relations firms to get news organizations on television, radio, newspapers, and magazines to do positive stories on their drugs. You'll notice when you're watching the news that many times there is a medical expert on who says something about a new drug. This medical expert never says it's his opinion, there is never an alternative viewpoint presented. The medical expert always gives the pro-drug side and it is presented as a news story. The fact is it is not news at all. The medical experts are in many cases spokespeople for the drug companies. These "medical experts" are being paid huge amounts of money to say all these wonderful things about drugs. Where is the full disclosure? When the news organization brings out their "medical expert," they never say, "By the way, our medical expert is being paid huge amounts of money to come on our show and say wonderful things about this drug." They are put on the news without any research whatsoever done by the news organization about whether the information itself being presented is factual, fair, balanced or honest. Everyone seems to forget that a new wonder drug makes billions of dollars in profits; and everyone seems to forget the drug companies are publicly traded companies and the people that own the stock in these companies have a major incentive for the drug company to sell more drugs. So the real question is: Who owns the stock in these drug companies? Would it surprise you that many members of the FDA and FTC own stock in drug companies? Would it surprise you that many members of Congress own stock in drug companies? Would it also surprise you that members of the news media that are supposed to be impartially presenting news own stock in drug companies? And the corporations that own television networks, radio networks, newspapers, and magazines all have financial ties to the pharmaceutical industry and all have incentives for the drug industry to sell more drugs?

That's one of the reasons why you hear so much about drugs on the news and read so many positive articles about drugs in magazines and newspapers. These organizations get financial benefit from the drugs that are sold. Additionally, most news organizations do not research the accuracy and truthfulness of information when presenting news about drugs. When they get a press release from the pharmaceutical industry, it is read and presented as news without question.

The pharmaceutical industry has an automatic outlet to get billions of dollars in free advertising which is being disguised as news. Doesn't it surprise you that on the news the only medical experts giving any information about health, illness, disease, or sickness are all medical doctors? And that the only information we are hearing is about the use of drugs? Doesn't it surprise you that you virtually never hear any positive news at all about an herbal remedy, a natural remedy, or a homeopathic remedy? Could it be that there is no profit in those remedies? Remember, natural remedies can not be patented.

The unholy alliance between the FDA, the FTC, and the drug industry created an interesting set of laws that magically appeared. The FDA and the FTC have the ability to make a law without it having to get passed through a vote in Congress. One of the laws that the FDA passed was this outrageous and totally irresponsible dictum: *The FDA has stated as law that the only thing that can cure or prevent a disease is a drug!*

Now why is this so outrageous? What the FDA has now determined is that there is absolutely no natural remedy that can cure or prevent any disease. Because if a natural remedy did, then it has to be classified as a "drug" and once it's classified as a drug it has to go through the $800 million worth of testing that the FDA requires to be approved as a new drug. This can not be done. Why? Because a natural remedy can not be patented and there is no company that can spend $800 million to get a natural remedy approved as a new drug because it will not own a patent for that "new drug" and therefore can't make that money back plus ten-fold profits. Natural remedies can not be patented. Therefore, it can not go through the testing that the FDA requires. This is why the FDA and drug companies love this system. It prevents any natural remedy from being touted as a cure or prevention of disease when in fact many of them are. The FDA has colluded with the drug industry and given the drug industry a monopoly.

Think about it. The FDA states that only a drug can cure or prevent a disease, absolutely nothing else can. How insane is that? To make matters worse, what the pharmaceutical industry and the FDA have done now is decided to classify more and more things as diseases. Once upon a time, you used to get heartburn, now it's called Acid Reflux Disease. Once upon a time people used to be shy, now it's classified as Social Anxiety Disorder, which is a disease. Kids who are eating too much sugar or are a little rambunctious are now classified as having attention deficit disorder, which is a disease. If a woman has a low sexual desire, it is now classified as a disease. An alcoholic is no longer an alcoholic; he now has the disease of alcoholism. A person who is overweight is no longer overweight they now have the disease of obesity. A male who can not get an erection is said to have a disease.

The reason more and more things are being classified as diseases is, once it is classified as a disease, legally there can be no natural, inexpensive remedy that can cure or prevent it. The FDA says only a drug can do that. The FDA has the final word on what is a "disease." Once the FDA has decided with final authority that something is a disease, any company making a claim that an all-natural product could possibly cure or prevent that disease can be legally entered by the FDA unannounced—with federal agents, guns drawn—and seize the natural product. The FDA can then shut that business down and put the people who are in charge of that business in jail for practicing medicine without a license or selling drugs without a license, even though they are not selling drugs at all, they could be selling something as benign as bread. This actually happened back in the 1970s when a gentleman named Ben Suarez sold bread that had a high fiber content. It was an all-natural bread that was high in fiber. He stated that eating a high fiber diet could potentially lower the risk of certain cancers. At the time that statement was not "proven." But because he made that statement, he was now, according to the FDA, selling a drug without a license. He wasn't selling a drug, he was selling bread. The FDA came in, seized the bread, and destroyed it. It was enough bread to feed a million homeless people. He offered to give the bread away to homeless people. The FDA said no, and the bread was destroyed. How sick! And why was it destroyed? Because he was selling an all-natural product, and was potentially tapping into the profits of one of the most powerful, profitable industries in the world. It's all about the money!

Websites: The pharmaceutical industry is doing a brilliant job producing all kinds of informational websites which appear to be consumer oriented, unbiased websites which give information to consumers about various illnesses, diseases, and cures. But the fact is these are not unbiased websites. It's a trick, it's a scam. These websites are paid for and put out by the drug industry. They are made to look and appear as if they are unbiased and are there to give information to the consumer and to protect the consumer. The fact of the matter is they are nothing more than websites owned directly or indirectly by the pharmaceutical companies to sell you more drugs.

Paying of Celebrities: This shocked me when I found this out. When you watch a TV talk show, or listen to talk radio, many times a celebrity is being interviewed. That celebrity may have had some kind of disease or a family member of that celebrity may have had some kind of disease. That celebrity is on that talk show talking about the particular disease that he or a family member or friends have suffered from, and they may talk about a new treatment that they've tried or a new drug that they've tried that cured them of the problem and saved their life and how wonderful it is. It sounds oh so interesting and oh so wonderful. It appears that this celebrity is genuinely concerned about the health and welfare of other people because they went through it in their personal life. But upon further investigation we find that these celebrities, most of whom are professional actors, are doing a brilliant job of acting, because they are being paid huge amounts of money by the drug industry to tout the drug company's drug under the disguise of a normal interview. These real talk shows are becoming infomercials for the drug industry. But you and I watch them and don't know they are in fact commercials. This celebrity, under the banner of full disclosure, never says that he is being paid huge amounts of money by the drug industry to tout the drug in public. Does this surprise you? It shouldn't, because it is common in every industry. A golf club manufacturer says "more tour professionals use our driver than any other brand." When interviewed, the tour professionals say how much they love their driver. What you are not told is that these golfers are paid millions of dollars to use the company's particular driver. So do we really know if the golfers are using this driver because it's the best driver, or are they using the driver because they are being paid to? Remember, it's always about the money.

Another technique that the drug industry uses to make sure sales of drugs continue to increase is to get the federal government to pass laws requiring people to take drugs. There are three methods employed. First, pass a law requiring that children must take a certain drug, such as vaccines. Second, pass a law requiring all federal employees and military personnel to take a certain drug. (Note the recent drives to have government employees and members of the military vaccinated against anthrax and smallpox.) Third, get the government to pay for drug usage for the poor and elderly through Social Security, Medicare, and Medicaid. When this happens…Bam! Billions of dollars in profits.

Remember the Anthrax scare in Washington? I believe it was a brilliant campaign to increase the sales of a certain antibiotic, Cipro. When the Anthrax scare went on the air, the drug companies did a brilliant marketing campaign talking about how Cipro is the drug of choice for Anthrax. Overnight the sales of Cipro skyrocketed. Millions of dollars in profits were generated by the drug companies.

- **Use of Books:** Drug companies pay millions of dollars to doctors, alleged experts, who are in fact paid directly or indirectly from the drug industry and are in fact paid spokespeople for the drug companies. These experts then write books about the health benefits of certain drugs. Go into any bookstore and you can see book after book after book promoting drug use by "an independent medical expert." The fact is the drug companies are paying the expert to write the books. The book is nothing more than an ad for the drug.

Among other methods used by the government in tandem with the drug industry:

- **Censorship of Opposing Ideas.** This is scary. We live in America. It's supposed to be the land of free speech. Well, speech is not free. If your speech happens to threaten the profits of big business, you are going to be bound and gagged, ridiculed and persecuted. Here's what happens:

There are hundreds of books written about the drug industry, the FDA, the FTC, and the collusion between the associations, the corporations, the lobbyists, and certain government regulators and how they work together to suppress all-natural, inexpensive ways to prevent and cure disease. These books and these authors never see the light of day. Why? Publishers won't publish these books. If a publisher publishes a book that is bashing the pharmaceutical industry, certain government agencies, or big business, the publishing company may be black-listed and have its other books taken out of distribution. Publishing companies fear that the publishing of these books will in fact cost them millions of dollars in profits. Additionally, many of the officers and directors of these publishing companies own stock in many pharmaceutical companies, and they do not want to do anything that will adversely affect their own personal portfolio. Remember, it's all about the money!

There is also censorship of advertising. Think about this very simply. Let's say that you are the president of a major television network. The particular network that you are the president of is owned by another multinational company that owns or has huge controlling interest in a drug company. Your network gets two-thirds, or close to 70 percent, of its advertising revenue directly from the drug industry. Now imagine a guy comes to you and says, "I'd like to advertise on your network my book entitled *How the Drug Companies Are Ripping Off America.*" Would you, as the president of that company, run that ad? If you run that ad, your boss could fire you. Because by running that ad, you could have a negative impact on the sales and profits of the drug companies in which your boss has a major equity position. That means it is costing your boss money. You may in fact own stock yourself. Think about it this way: If you run that ad for that book, how are your other advertisers going to feel? What if they called you up and said "Hey, if you run that ad for that book, we're not going to run any of our drug ads next month." Your sales are going to go straight down and you'll probably be fired. Folks, this is what is happening. It's all about the money.

- **Debunking Natural Remedies.** In an actual government memorandum, the U.S. federal government states that one of the most effective tools to get people to believe the government's opinion is to put together a well orchestrated debunking campaign. What this means is there is a coordinated effort between the FDA, the FTC, the healthcare associations, and the entire pharmaceutical industry—as well as some major news organizations—to produce scare stories about natural alternatives and suppress the truth about the ineffectiveness and dangers of drugs. There is a long list of inexpensive, highly effective natural cures that are being labeled as "snake oil" or simply hidden from the public.

The FDA has led the way in this battle against natural cures. In the 1970s the FDA attempted to make vitamin supplements prescription drugs. The FDA claimed that vitamins are so dangerous they should be prescribed only by doctors. The public was outraged and Congress rejected the idea. In 1993 the FDA tried to classify certain minerals and amino acids as prescription drugs. Again, a public outcry caused Congress to act. Recently the FDA has been going after companies that sell natural remedies via the Internet. It claims these companies are selling "drugs" without a license.

In the book *The Assault on Medical Freedom,* secret documents from the medical industry have been exposed proving the FDA, the pharmaceutical industry, the AMA, and even insurance companies are working together to discredit natural medicine. The documents show how the FDA worked with the pharmaceutical industry directly, producing the "public service, anti-quackery campaign" which is designed to make people believe alternative natural remedies are ineffective, a waste of money, and even harmful. This "public service campaign" is simply a front of the pharmaceutical industry. The author claims that this collusion between the government and the pharmaceutical industry has created "nothing less than an enforced totalitarian medical-pharmaceutical police state."

The FDA targets natural remedies one at a time. Their debunking campaign begins by warning the public that these substances have not been properly tested, are potentially dangerous and should not be used. Even when double blind studies prove the effectiveness or safety of the remedies, the evidence is debunked, suppressed, or ignored.

There are thousands of studies that prove not only that natural remedies are effective, but they can be more effective than any drug counterpart. An example is Vitamin E. In major double blind studies, Vitamin E was found as effective or more effective as a blood thinner than its drug counterpart. But why aren't we given Vitamin E instead of the drug? The facts are clear: Natural remedies could financially devastate the pharmaceutical industry.

Virtually every day we hear about "warnings" relating to the usage of dietary supplements. The news organizations that report this information, for the most part, do virtually no research into the accuracy or truthfulness of these warnings. There are different standards used in what is classified as news and advertising. If information is presented by a politician or government agency, such as the FDA or FTC, news organizations present that information as 100 percent factual. Any press release submitted to a news reporting organization by a politician or government agency is reported as 100 percent fact. The news reporting agency rarely if ever investigates the claims or allegations, or seeks out an opposing viewpoint. The government has the ability to influence the masses at will without opposition. So, the first standard set is that anything a government agency or politician says is true and evidence is not required to support their claims.

The next standard set is for "big business." When large publicly traded corporations send out press releases to news organizations, very little verification is done on the accuracy and truthfulness of what is presented. The information is reported as news, but because it is coming from business and not the government, occasionally opposing viewpoints are presented as well.

The FTC allows big business to do things in their advertising that smaller businesses would be prohibited from doing. Example: You are watching an ad on television. At the bottom of the screen there are several lines of "disclaimers." The FTC requires that these disclaimers be present. However, because it's big business, they are allowed to put the disclaimers on the screen for just a few seconds, and printed so small there is not a human being in the world who can read them! It's an absolute joke.

Additionally, big business ads are allowed to do something that small advertisers are routinely prosecuted for. If a small advertiser, let's say a company selling a piece of exercise equipment through a TV infomercial, were to have a man dressed up as a doctor making wonderful statements about the product, that man must be a doctor, can not be a paid spokesperson, and must not be reading a script. However, in big business advertising when you see doctors, judges, business executives, policemen etc., making statements about how wonderful the company's products are, you are being deceived and lied to. These people are paid actors reading a script! If a small company selling a product on an infomercial did the same thing they would be shut down and prosecuted for false and misleading advertising. The bottom line is the government and politicians can say anything on TV, and it is never challenged and it is presented as 100 percent truth. Big business can do almost anything on TV and produce false and misleading advertising without the FTC preventing them.

Small businesses or companies threatening the profits of "big business" are the ones routinely attacked by the FTC, the FDA and other regulatory agencies. It is surprising to note that the majority of actions taken by the FTC and FDA are against small and medium sized businesses. They rarely if ever go after big business. For example, the FTC's Field Manual states that agents should not go after "big business" because they have deep pockets and will fight back against the FTC. It instructs its agents not to go after very small businesses because they have no money. It states to go after medium sized businesses that will settle quickly out of fear. It's shocking to note that the Federal Trade Commission does not take action against companies based on consumer complaints, but rather uses political pressure on who to go after and the amount of money that can be extracted from the company.

Did you know that when the FTC charges a company with false and misleading advertising and then collects money for "consumer redress," it never gives the money to the consumer? The FTC keeps the money! This agency is supposed to protect the consumers, yet the vast majority of actions filed by the FTC are against companies where there are no consumer complaints. The FTC and the FDA work together to spread misinformation and lies about all-natural remedies. Think of the millions of dollars that are poured into public relations campaigns specifically designed to debunk and make natural remedies appear foolish. So-called consumer advocate associations, or watchdog groups, have sprung up with fancy names that sound like they are looking out to protect the consumer when in fact these particular organizations are nothing more than a front for the pharmaceutical industry to promote their products, increase drug usage, and increase the nation's perception that natural remedies don't work and are dangerous.

A good example of this is Ephedra. Ephedra is a compound most commonly found in the herb mahuang. This herb has been used for centuries around the world, most notably in China, as a very effective herbal remedy for various types of illness including obesity and asthma. It is safe and incredibly effective. Ephedra was a substance used in diet aids to increase metabolism and decrease appetite. It did an outstanding job. If you took massive amounts and did not follow the instructions on the bottle, you may have had some adverse effects, such as nervousness or the jitters similar to drinking twenty cups of coffee. In a very well orchestrated debunking campaign, the FDA has banned the use of Ephedra stating it is dangerous. This was a very coordinated effort to get people to believe that a natural herbal supplement could be dangerous. This campaign is designed to encourage Congress to ban more natural remedies, as well as require supplements as harmless as basic vitamins and minerals to be classified as drugs and be sold by prescription and manufactured by the pharmaceutical industry. This is being touted under the guise of safety. Safety has nothing to do with it. Why?

Ephedra was banned because 153 deaths have been linked to taking Ephedra. Now, millions of people were taking Ephedra. If you take any group of ten million people, over a year, there's a good chance that 153 people in that group will die. The FDA said there is a "link" between Ephedra use and those deaths. There is absolutely no conclusive evidence that Ephedra caused those deaths or even had any remote association with those deaths. However, the FDA keeps saying how dangerous Ephedra is. Every single nonprescription drug is dangerous! If you went into your medicine cabinet, took a drug, and took more than what the label said, there is a high probability that you could die. Every single drug is incredibly dangerous. This is not about danger, it is about who controls these products. The scary part is whatever the FDA says, it is presented as truth and no opposing opinions are allowed to be heard.

Think about this. Two thousand people died simply by taking aspirin. Not overdosing on aspirin, but by taking aspirin in the recommended amounts. Wow! It appears that aspirin is not safe. Yet, I don't see aspirin being banned. Do you see where this is going? This debunking campaign includes two things: getting news organizations and various publications to do positive stories about drugs, falsifying or misrepresenting research data on drugs, while at the same time spreading any type of negative information about a natural remedy and natural holistic healers.

Another perfect example of this debunking campaign was a headline that said "Saint John's Wort Not Effective for Treating Depression, Study Concludes." The article—written in a national newspaper—stated that a recent study was conducted and proved that Saint John's Wort, the herbal remedy touted as a depression alleviant, was found to have absolutely no effect on depression. This article went on to talk about how many herbs are used to treat various illnesses and disease without any research whatsoever to back up the effectiveness of those herbs. The article then went on to state that people should not take any herbs or natural substances because they could be unsafe and are probably ineffective.

The article was ridiculous, one-sided and outrageous. Why do I say that? Because when you actually look at that particular study they were referring to, Saint John's Wort was tested in addition to Prozac in the exact same study. And the study showed that Prozac and Saint John's Wort both had no effect on depression in the patients in the study. But the news organization never mentioned that Prozac was also proven to be ineffective. It also failed to mention that there are dozens of studies that show that Saint John's Wort is, in fact, effective. But obviously this study was flawed. The fact is that you can create a study to show virtually anything you want, but the news media chose only to talk negatively about the herbal, all-natural supplement and didn't have anything negative to say about the drug. Debunking by use of studies is very common. Most "studies" are funded by the drug industry. The researchers are given very specific parameters and objectives. Since these studies are funded by the pharmaceutical industry, the objectives are to show that drugs are effective and safe, and all-natural treatments are ineffective and dangerous. These researchers are given financial incentives to produce these results: millions of dollars in additional grants, funding, future contracts, as well as luxury perks like vacations and cars. Imagine how this works. Any research results a pharmaceutical company wants, it can get; all it has to do is buy it!

Here's an example, parents were concerned that their children were eating too much sugar, causing hyperactivity, learning disabilities and behavioral problems. The sugar industry was concerned that kids would be eating less sugar, thus cutting into their profits. (Remember the role of the food companies in all this, from our discussion at the beginning of the chapter.) The sugar industry associations indirectly funded a study, which was to prove that sugar consumption had no effect on hyperactivity or learning abilities. They got the study with the results they wanted. In a national newspaper, the headline read: "Sugar Has No Effect on Hyperactivity or Learning and Behavioral Problems in Children." The article stated that a study was conducted with two groups of children. The first group was given a "controlled diet." The second group ate the exact same controlled diet, but 30 percent more sugar. The hyperactivity level, learning abilities and behavioral actions were found to be the same in both groups. This concluded that sugar did not increase hyperactivity or cause learning or behavioral problems in children.

Here is what they didn't tell you. The study had only ten children in it, five in each group! Certainly not enough to have any accuracy on the study results. (This happens routinely. Studies are conducted with just a few people just so the results the companies need can be achieved.) Secondly, you were not told that the controlled diet contained lots of sugar in it. It actually contained enormous amounts of sugar. The controlled diet contained the sugar equivalent of eating twenty-five doughnuts, drinking three dozen sodas, and eating ten candy bars. So all the kids were so hyped up on sugar that when you added 30 percent more, there wasn't any change! Can you see how out-rageous this is? Can you see you are being lied to and misled? Can you see why I'm mad as hell and not going to take it anymore? I can give you dozens of examples of studies that simply are false and misleading. You can create any "credible scientific evidence" you want if you just pay the right people.

Drugs are not the answer for the prevention and curing of disease. Natural methods work better in the long term, and are much safer than drugs and surgery. "They" don't want you to know the truth. "They" use television, radio, newspapers and magazines, including the use of paid celebrities, paid experts, and false and misleading advertising to convince you that drugs are good and natural remedies are bad.

- **Lawsuits.** The industry uses lawsuits as a tool to spread negative information about natural remedies and also to put out of business anyone that is challenging the profits of the pharmaceutical indus-try. Keep in mind the pharmaceutical industry is the most powerful, profitable business in the world.

Some of you remember the movie *The Fugitive*. Well, that was more fact than fiction. Some of you may remember that the whole reason Dr. Kimble, played by Harrison Ford, was found guilty of murdering his wife was because a doctor was falsifying research on a new drug and stood to make tens of million of dollars if the drug was approved by the FDA. Folks I can tell you that happens! It's scary but true. The industry has so much money, has such deep pockets, they can afford to file outrageous, frivolous lawsuits against small independent people and companies, and virtually drive them out of business or bring them to their knees.

One particular case was with the American Medical Association. Keep in mind the AMA is a union for its members, not a government organi-zation with the mandate of solving the medical problems of America. The American Medical Association has no interest in you and me, we are simply customers. The American Medical Association is a union designed to protect its members which are the medical doctors and the medical industry. But it is always being presented as an independent, unbiased body presenting medical facts to the world, with a goal of cur-ing disease, which simply is not the case. Just read their charter.

The history of the AMA is fascinating. The AMA was founded in 1847 in Philadelphia. While there were many state medical associations at the time, the need to establish a national association that would look after the interests of medical doctors nationwide was determined to be paramount one year earlier at the New York medical convention. At the time, doctors were not the majority of heathcare practitioners in America dealing with the cure and prevention of illness and disease. There were vast amounts of homeopathic and other practitioners using natural remedies. The very next year after being created, the AMA began its organized assault on debunking natural remedies and discrediting any healthcare practitioner who was not a medical doctor. At the same time it set out to establish the laws governing patent medicine. This practice has continued ever since, thus establishing the healthcare monopoly for the medical doctor as these continued to expand into the areas of drug manufacturing and medical research. Today, the American Medical Association stands as the largest and most powerful healthcare association in the world. It has amassed enough power and influence to create laws that help expand the business of its members while at the same time eliminating any competition that might threaten their outrageous profits.

From this position of power, the AMA filed a lawsuit against the chiropractors in Illinois. Chiropractors at the time were saying that chiropractic adjustments can alleviate pain. Many people were going to chiropractors instead of medical doctors. The AMA, in order to protect its members, filed a lawsuit against the chiropractors. The chiropractors fought back, and fought back big time. The chiropractors won. It was proven in court that chiropractic treatments were better at eliminating or reducing pain than anything that medical doctors could offer. But the travesty is that the case got almost no press at all. Can you see why? That was a huge landmark case but got virtually no press whatsoever.

Another huge case which got virtually no press whatsoever was when a doctor, who was treating people through all-natural methods, was saying that his all-natural nondrug methods were curing people of AIDS. He was immediately sued by the FDA. The case went all the way to the New York Supreme Court and the doctor was found not guilty. It was proven that his treatments were more effective than those offered by any medical doctor, and he was using no drugs or surgery, only all-natural methods. Did you read about this in the newspapers? Of course not. Did you hear about it on any of the TV news stations or radio news stations? No. Did you read about it in any major front page articles in magazines? Absolutely not. Remember, it's all about the money.

Lawsuits are routinely filed against individual healthcare practitioners who are curing people without drugs or surgery. Not only civil lawsuits filed against them, but many of these honest, dedicated, healthcare providers are being prosecuted criminally for curing people's diseases. They are being charged with practicing medicine without a license or dispensing drugs without a license. Their only real crime is curing disease through natural methods and not using drugs and surgery. Lawsuits are also routinely filed against companies that sell all-natural products that can prevent or cure diseases. These lawsuits are filed primarily by the FTC, the FDA, and watchdog groups, which are really fronts for the pharmaceutical industry and medical associations. These suits are filed even though there are no consumer complaints! Remember, when these lawsuits are filed, the allegations are presented as facts by the news media. Also remember that virtually all television networks, radio networks, newspapers and magazines depend on the advertising revenue they receive from the pharmaceutical industry. What you read about and what you hear about will always be influenced by the pharmaceutical industry.

These attacks via lawsuit are increasing at an alarming rate. Recently the FDA, the FTC, and several other government agencies have teamed up and launched a campaign called "Operation Cure All." The reason this campaign has been launched is said to be to protect the health of consumers against natural products that are not proven effective or safe. These government agencies are making the playing field uneven. Operation Cure All allows the pharmaceutical industry to produce their deceptive and false advertising, while at the same time setting strict rules as to what is truthful, substantiated, and allowable in advertising for natural health products. One rule is the prohibition on saying that a natural product does anything relating to the prevention or curing of a disease. Not only are you prohibited from making such a statement, even if it is true; you are forbidden to *imply* such a claim.

The amazing thing is that the courts have determined that the FTC has the authority to decide whether a claim is implied or not. This means the FTC has the absolute final word on whether an ad is in violation of law. This ultimately means that the FTC can at any time sue a company or individual, and they will always win.

Under the banner of Operation Cure All, telling the truth is also forbidden. A person is prohibited from telling what the product has done for him, even though his statement may be 100 percent truthful and accurate. The FTC and the FDA have effectively taken over the right of free speech under the guise of protecting the public. Why are drug companies allowed to advertise their products on television, on radio, and in newspapers and magazines so freely? These ads are clearly false and misleading. The testimonials you hear are fake. You are watching paid actors who are reading a script. You are being lied to and deceived and both the FDA and FTC take no action. Why is it that advertising for natural products are being routinely attacked? It is obvious to everyone that the truth about natural remedies is being suppressed.

How can America, a country that presents itself to the world as a bastion of free speech, free expression of ideas, freedom of choice, freedom of information and free enterprise, be faced with such draconian restrictions of these freedoms when it relates to our health and medical choices? Operation Cure All is part of a new set of rules being implemented to restrict and limit access to health information, food supplements, and natural therapies on a worldwide basis. The World Health Organization, the United Nations, international banks, and the multinational pharmaceutical industry are working together right now, implementing these regulations. This worldwide commission is working on restrictions that would severely limit the availability of vitamins, food supplements, natural remedies and even information.

It appears the actual objective of this organization is to bring natural dietary supplements under the umbrella of the pharmaceutical industry. Is it true that the pharmaceutical industry is trying to take over all-natural products? In America, pharmaceutical giants are buying vitamin, mineral, herbal, and homeopathic companies. Currently there are two products being marketed on television. The ads look eerily similar to drug ads. The packaging of the products makes them appear to be drugs. But in this instance, they are not drugs at all. They are natural products being manufactured and sold by the pharmaceutical industry at outrageous prices, because it's the pharmaceutical industry, these ads are allowed to run. If a small, independent company were running the same ad, the FTC would come in and charge them with false and misleading advertising, and making unsubstantiated health claims. The FDA would come in, seize the product, confiscate the equipment, books, records and computers of the company, and charge the officers, directors and owners with selling drugs without a license. I know this to be true because I actually transcribed these ads, changed a couple of words and presented them to both the FTC and FDA. I asked if these ads would violate any of the FTC or FDA rules. I was told that these ads violated both FTC and FDA rules and regulations. Hmm. Imagine their surprise when I informed them that these ads were being run by big pharmaceutical companies. Their response was "we'll look into it." But they assured me that if I ran these ads action would be taken against me immediately. We are supposed to have equal protection under the law. Selective prosecution is allegedly forbidden in this country. Unfortunately, that's not how it works. The bottom line here is that the government is working together with the pharmaceutical industry to take control of all-natural remedies. For example, in Germany and Norway the drug companies have virtually taken over the entire health food industry. Vitamin B1, Vitamin C and Vitamin E, in certain amounts, are illegal in these countries. A major pharmaceutical company now controls the herb Echinacea, and sells it as an over-the-counter drug at exorbitant prices. Selling herbs as food, in certain parts of Europe, is now a criminal offense.

Am I the only voice expressing outrage? No. There are thousands of medical doctors, scientists, surgeons, and ex-pharmaceutical insiders who know the truth and are desperately trying to educate the public. Hundreds of books have been written on these subjects; I am not the only one.

The bottom line is that there ARE natural, inexpensive, safe cures for almost every disease. The pharmaceutical industry, the FTC, the FDA and the rest of "them" are trying to suppress this information.

The pharmaceutical industry, the drug industry, the food industry, the associations and government agencies, all have a major financial incentive to keep people sick. There are billions of dollars in profits as long as people stay sick and there are billions of dollars in profits as long as people take more and more drugs. Remember, it's always about the money!

• • •

I have to blow the whistle on how the FTC and FDA operate. The Federal Trade Commission is an agency with the primary goal of protecting consumers. It was formed to guard consumers against monopolies, and ensure that small businesses were given a level playing field within which to operate. The FTC's other main goal is to make sure that consumers are not "ripped off" by companies. Yet in actual fact, the FTC has no interest in protecting consumers.

Let me give you an example from my own personal experience. This is not an isolated case. I can show you hundreds of examples proving that this is in fact the standard operating procedure of the FTC. Here is what it looks like:

I was excited about a product called coral calcium. This product is simply calcium, the source being coral sand from Okinawa, Japan. Calcium is harmless, has many proven health benefits, is an essential nutrient for the body, and has been sold for years without any issues.

I produced a TV infomercial interviewing an author who was giving his **opinions** about the potential health benefits of supplementing your diet with calcium. I then sent this infomercial to the FTC. I telephoned the FTC on several occasions. I wrote the FTC several letters. I sent several e-mails. I kept asking the FTC if they had any issues with my television commercial promoting the product coral calcium. I informed the FTC that if there were any concerns or questions they needed answered, to please communicate that to me as my intention and desire was to be 100 percent cooperative in every way.

The FTC responded on several occasions that they had no issues with my promotion of coral calcium. The coral calcium product was being embraced by the public. Thousands of letters kept pouring in telling of the incredible health benefits people were experiencing from taking coral calcium. The return rate of the product was one of the lowest in the entire dietary supplement industry. There were virtually no complaints, and everyone seemed to like coral calcium. Unbeknownst to me, the FTC was conducting a secret investigation into the sale and promotion of coral calcium, and were coordinating their efforts with the FDA. During the entire investigation, the FTC never called us or requested any information from us at all.

Suddenly, without warning, the FTC filed a major lawsuit against me, my company, and the author I interviewed. The lawsuit stated that we were making unsubstantiated health claims about the benefits of coral calcium. They went to court and asked for an emergency ruling demanding that the company be shut down, and all of my personal assets frozen.

This is the *modus operandi* of the FTC.

First, they conduct a secret investigation. No matter how cooperative you want to be, they refuse to talk to or question the company or individual that they are getting ready to pounce on. Secondly, they go into court and demand that the companies be shut down and all assets frozen. Unbelievable as it sounds, the FTC wins this request over 97 percent of the time. The opposing side is given virtually no time to respond and is, in effect, put out of business. It may also surprise you to know that when the FTC files suit, it is not required to go to federal court. Instead, the FTC suits are presented before an "administrative law judge" who is actually an employee of the FTC! The "courtroom" is in the FTC building itself! No wonder the FTC wins 97 percent of the time. Further research revealed that, with the exception of a few antitrust cases involving huge companies, not one single administrative judge ever ruled against the FTC.

My case is almost identical to most other FTC cases. The three most outrageous things to look at are:

1. The FTC stated that we were making unsubstantiated and false health claims about coral calcium. However, how could the FTC

make that allegation when they **never** asked us to produce any substantiation that we may have had? Making the allegation without asking us or reviewing the substantiation that we had is in itself a false and misleading statement. The FTC is guilty of making false and misleading statements and then presenting them to the media as facts.

2. Where are all the complaining customers? If our advertising was so deceptive, customers would have complained and returned the product. The FTC's response to this is that the public is too stupid to know that the ad violated the FTC rules.

3. Why didn't the FTC contact us or respond to our multitude of letters, phone calls and e-mails? For over a year and a half, the FTC knew about our ad. We repeatedly asked them if they had any issues. They repeatedly said no. Then the sudden lawsuit, and the subsequent demand that the show be pulled off the air. Why the delay? This is standard operating procedure. If the FTC really thought that our infomercial was not fair to consumers, they could have asked us to take it off the air eighteen months earlier. Why did they wait? Because it's all about the money! The FTC routinely waits for companies to generate large amounts of sales and profits before they step in and take action. They do this because they do not care about the consumer, all they want is money. If they stopped you right in the beginning you wouldn't have any money to give them.

Why Are We Sick?

Health is a state of complete physical, mental, and social well-being, and not merely the absence of disease and infirmity. —**World Health Organization**

We spend more money on healthcare than ever before. We take more drugs than ever before, yet we are sicker than ever before. More people are getting sick than ever before in history. As I mentioned in the beginning of this book, there are no such things as medical facts. Everything is simply an opinion based on the information we have at the current time. Additionally, all "medical facts" that are presented are those opinions which make the most profits. If information about the prevention, cure or diagnosis of disease was found to have an adverse effect on publicly traded companies' profits (primarily the pharmaceutical industry and the medical industry), then that "medical fact" will not be presented at all, it will be debunked and it will be suppressed.

There is an underground movement which includes hundreds of thousands of healthcare practitioners who treat patients every day and see people get healed every single day. These healthcare practitioners do not use drugs or surgery, they use all-natural methods. The individual patients who are cured know that these all-natural treatments work. There are no complaints lodged with any government agency. Yet the FDA and other government agencies are on a mission to stamp out and wipe out all of these natural healthcare practitioners. Why? Because they cut into the profits of the drug companies.

Over the years, the pharmaceutical industry has come up with different theories about why people get sick. First it was bacteria and germs. The super wonder drug of the day was antibiotics, which were touted as the method that would eliminate disease forever and cure all illness, sickness and diseases. The theory was that all disease was caused by germs, primarily bacteria. This theory has proved to be wrong. Stronger and stronger antibiotics are continually developed, yet people continue to get sicker, and sicker, and sicker. More people are getting more diseases than ever before.

The next theory was that viruses were the cause of all illness and disease. Unfortunately, few people know that antibiotics have no effect on viruses. The doctors continually prescribe antibiotics at the drop of a hat. People have been brainwashed into thinking that antibiotics are needed when they feel sick, and go to their doctors and demand antibiotics. The doctor, who unfortunately is in a business and understands his patient is really a customer, has to make the customer happy and prescribes the antibiotic. If the doctor does not, the patient (aka, the customer) will simply find another doctor who will prescribe an antibiotic. The Associated Press reported that overuse of broad-spectrum of antibiotics for minor infection poses a serious health threat. The government estimates that half of the one hundred million antibiotic prescriptions written each year are totally unnecessary. Still, people continue to get more diseases, more sickness and more illness.

The current theory of the day is all sickness, diseases, and illnesses are caused by genetic defects. Of course the only answer is drugs. Drugs are now being researched and looked at to handle these genetic defects. The new method of making billions of dollars in profit is to come up with a genetic defect for every problem a person has. We hear it every day, "Oh, you're fat because you have a genetic defect, and a drug is being worked on that can solve that genetic defect and make you thin." "Diabetes is nothing more than genetics, so we'll work on a drug that will correct that genetic disposition and solve the problem." Keep in mind that drug companies really do not want to cure disease as they claim. If they came up with a cure, they would be out of business.

Think of herpes. Herpes is a virus. We hear ads on TV every day that say "There is no cure for herpes"; therefore, in order to suppress the symptoms, take our beautiful, wonderful drug every day for the rest of your life. Imagine what would happen to the publicly traded company and their stock price if they announced "Here is a cure for herpes, simply take this herb for thirty days and you will never have a herpetic breakout ever again. By the way, this herb is not patented and it only costs three dollars." That company would lose billions of dollars in profits and valuation. Its stock price would plummet. Therefore, there is no incentive to cure herpes. The incentive is to keep you brainwashed into believing there is no cure for herpes, and the only solution to the "symptoms" is drugs. Remember, the FDA and the drug companies work hand in hand. If I happen to know a cure for herpes, I can not say so. Because if I say so I am now making a medical claim and, according to the FDA, I am now breaking the law. Even if what I am saying is true, I am still breaking the law. The FDA will then come in with their federal agents with their guns drawn, arrest me, throw me in jail, confiscate any papers I have (and any of the harmless herb), suppress the information and outlaw it because there is no "credible scientific evidence." They will then put out press releases and statements of "fact" that I am a charlatan selling snake oil and have no scientific evidence to substantiate that what I am saying is true. Unfortunately, that's how the system works.

Later in this book I will tell you how we are going to change the system by blowing the whistle on the pharmaceutical industry, the FDA, the FTC, the crooked charities and foundations, the associations, and the politicians. I am going to name names and expose the individual people whose identities have been kept a secret up until now. Isn't it strange that you are never informed of the identity of the directors or major shareholders of these organizations? These individual people hide behind corporations, trusts and a maze of legal structures so that their true identities remain hidden. If the money trail were followed, it would shock you to find that it leads to a small group of billionaires from around the world that are truly pulling the strings. Through class action lawsuits and a grassroots campaign, we will get the truth out about healthcare. The trend will reverse, drug use will go down and people will stop getting sick.

So why do you get sick? Is it germs? Is it bacteria? Is it viruses? Is it genetics? Well let's think about it. You don't catch cancer. Your body develops cancer. You don't catch diabetes. Your body develops diabetes. You don't catch obesity. Your body becomes fat and obese. You don't catch heartburn or acid reflux, as it is called today. It's developed. You don't catch headaches, you don't catch fibromyalgia, you don't catch back pain, you don't catch arthritis, you don't catch PMS and you don't catch impotence. These are all "medical conditions" that are developed in the body. You don't catch them. It's not a germ. It's not a virus. It's not bacteria. The majority of illness is in fact self-inflicted. Drugs are not the answer. You don't have a headache because you have an aspirin deficiency. The question is, why do human beings have so much illness?

First of all you have to realize that being sick is not normal and it is not the natural state of the body. Your body is not supposed to get sick. Think about this startling fact. Animals don't get heart attacks. Let me say that again, animals **never** get heart attacks. Why do humans? Animals don't get cancer, diabetes, arthritis, or virtually any of the common human diseases. Animals virtually never get sick, except of course when they are in captivity. When animals are under human care and get vaccine injections, drugs, and human processed food, animals succumb to many of the diseases that humans are riddled with.

Think about this: Animals do not exercise and have no obesity or weight problem. Animals don't go to doctors and live to be ten to twenty times their maturity age. Chimpanzees and gorillas are great examples. They don't lose their teeth, they don't have arthritis, they don't have diabetes, they don't need insulin shots, they don't have cancer, they don't have asthma, they don't have allergies, they are not constipated, they don't have insomnia, and they live to be an equivalent of about 180 years old. Interestingly enough, they go through their entire lives without taking any prescription or non-prescription drug.

So is there a way that we as human beings can do some very simple and easy things that can keep us disease free, illness free and full of life, energy, and vitality? The answer is: absolutely yes! Let's go back to the cause of all disease and the reason why we are sick.

Think about the fact that there are cultures around the world where the people have never had cancer or heart disease, or acid reflux disease, or prostate problems, etc. Yet when these people start living a western lifestyle, amazing things begin to happen to their health. They get fat, they start getting sick, and they begin to develop all of the common diseases we hear about today. The question is: Why do human beings living a western lifestyle have more sickness and disease than other human beings around the globe? The answer is, no one **knows**! The medical industry presents information as if they do know. They claim they have "scientific evidence" proving the truth of their theories. The fact is, what the medical industry has are only **theories**. When you investigate what is being presented as fact, you find that they are actually only theories that are nothing more than the opinions of individual people. Einstein's theory of relativity is presented as a fact, but people forget it's called the **theory** of relativity and not the **fact** of relativity.

The term "scientific evidence" is one of the greatest deceptions of all time. First, this "scientific evidence" is paid for and manufactured by the corporations that it will benefit. Rarely does an independent, unbiased third party produce any of this "scientific evidence." If the "scientific evidence" is so accurate, why are the conclusions and results constantly being disproved when new research is produced? You are led to believe that "scientific evidence" proves that something is true. This is a false assumption. Every day we hear "new research shows old research to be false." The bottom line is, you will hear the term "scientifically proven" used when the medical community claims they know the cause of disease. You will hear medical doctors make statements of fact when, in reality, they are only opinions. You are being misled and you are being lied to. You are being deceived. The truth is nobody knows why people are getting so sick, we can only guess and come up with our own theories and conclusions.

So, based on personal experience, reading thousands of pages of documents, and hearing the firsthand accounts from thousands of people and healthcare practitioners around the world, I have come up with what I believe to be the cause of virtually all sickness and disease in the body.

There are only two reasons why a person becomes ill:

1. They "catch" something. This means your body picked up a "germ," generally a virus or bacteria.

2. You "develop" an illness or disease. This means there is some imbalance in the body, something is not working right, and an illness or disease develops. Common diseases in this category include heart disease, cancer, diabetes, acid reflux, arthritis, etc.

Remember, in our search for the ultimate cause of all illness and the ultimate cure for all illnesses, we must always ask the question "What caused **that**?" With this in mind, let's start with "catching something."

One may say that the "cause" of catching a germ is pretty evident. You obviously caught the germ from someone else who had it. This is where medical science stops. They claim that drugs must be developed to kill these bacteria and viruses. However, they are asking the wrong question. The fact is that we are all exposed to bacteria and viruses on a daily basis. If one person in your home or office has the flu, then every single person has been exposed to and "caught" the flu virus. When anthrax was found in the envelope, not every single person in that building got anthrax! The question is not whether you will pick up bacteria or a virus, the real question is why do some people succumb to the bacteria and virus and get sick, and other people do not?

Take two people. Expose them both to the flu virus at the same time. One person comes down with all of the symptoms of the flu and becomes very sick. The other person shows no symptoms whatsoever, stays healthy, and does not "get the flu." They both got the flu virus! One person succumbed to it and got sick; the other person did not and remained healthy. Throughout your life you will pick up thousands of bacteria and viruses. That is natural. The real question to ask is why your body does not do what it was designed to do: fight off and handle the bacteria or virus. Why did you succumb to the bacteria or virus?

The answer: Your body is out of balance and your immune system is weak. If your body was in balance, a state called homeostasis, and your immune system was strong, you would never show any symptoms of any of the viruses or bacteria that you pick up during your lifetime. **You would never get sick because of a virus or bacteria.** Then the question becomes, "What is causing my body to be out of balance, and what is causing my immune system to be weak?"

I will give you the answer in a moment, but first let's go to the second reason people get sick. Remember, you get sick because you either "catch something" or something develops in the body on its own. You "catch something" because your body is out of balance and your immune system is weak. You develop something in the body either because your body is out of balance, or a "toxin" is getting into your body and causing the problem to develop. So let's walk through this nice and slow.

The reasons you get sick are:

1. Your body is out of balance (which means it's not functioning normally).
2. Your immune system is weak (which means it's not functioning normally).
3. Toxins are getting into your body.

What is a toxin? A toxin is a poison. It is a substance that, if taken in large doses at one time, would cause severe illness or death. Now the question is: What causes the body to be out of balance? Answer: putting toxins in the body and not putting into the body enough of the "right stuff." What causes the immune system to be weak? Answer: putting toxins in the body and not putting enough of the "right stuff" into the body. Hmm, we seem to be making progress! It appears then that all illness is caused by two things:

1. Toxins being put into the body.
2. Not putting enough of the "right stuff" in the body.

Let's use our magic question: What caused that? In relation to toxins, the question is what is causing toxins to be put into our body? The answer is that we have not been educated to know what these toxins are. And secondly, these toxins are being put in virtually everything we eat without our knowledge. Now, here is the big one: The most toxic thing you can put in your body, and the number one cause of virtually all illness and disease, is prescription and nonprescription drugs!

In my opinion, probably the number one reason people are sick is because of the amount of drugs they take. The statistics show very conclusively that the more prescription and nonprescription drugs a person takes, the sicker they are. Why? Because all drugs have negative side effects. Let me say it again, all drugs have negative side effects! If you are taking a drug to suppress one symptom, that drug is causing some other major problem to start developing in your body. Even if you stop taking that drug, the wheels have been set in motion, and in a few weeks or a few months—boom—you have some more symptoms caused by the first drug you took a few months ago. You go to your doctor, and he gives you another drug to suppress these new symptoms. This new drug had negative side effects, and after you start taking it the wheels will have already been put in motion, and voila! You have new symptoms which were in fact caused by the drug you were just taking. You go to your doctor and he gives you another drug. Drugs cause medical problems!

Drugs only suppress symptoms, they do not treat the cause. It's a great business for the drug companies. If they get you taking one drug, man, they've got you. Because that drug is not only going to suppress the symptom, probably, it is also going to cause you to have another symptom in a very short period of time, for which you will be prescribed another drug. Once they get you to take one drug to suppress a symptom (keeping in mind that it is not addressing the cause anyway), the likelihood of you taking another drug, and then another drug, and then another drug, keeps going up, and up, and up. The more drugs you take, the sicker you get, simply because drugs are major poisons, drugs are major toxins. Someone says, "Drugs can't really be poison, can they?" Then why don't you take thirty of them right now and see what happens? You'll probably die! If you eat thirty apples you're not going to die. You may feel full, but you are not going to die. Think about it.

Now, I love it when somebody says, "Well, it's in such a small amount," referring to the dosage. What if I put the same amount of my urine in your food? Would you eat it? Of course not!

This is the big shocker. The industry that is promoting itself as the group dedicated to the prevention and cure of disease is actually the group causing more sickness and disease to occur than ever before. All drugs are chemicals. All drugs have negative side effects. All drugs can cause death. All drugs are poisons. An outstanding book, which I highly recommend that you read, is *Overdose: The Case Against the Drug Companies,* written by Dr. J. Cohen M.D. Did you know that 250,000 Americans die every year from a prescription or nonprescription drug? That over 2,000 people last year died from taking aspirin? That there are dozens of articles showing how prescription and nonprescription drugs are **causing** all illness and diseases. Drugs are not the answer to preventing and curing disease. They are the cause! Even if drugs do not directly cause a disease, drugs cause the body to go completely out of balance, and they weaken the immune system so that diseases become more prevalent. People who get sick the most often are those who have taken the most drugs.

Let's back up just for a moment. Our conclusion is that all illness is caused by two things, one being the toxins in the body. When you have lots of toxins in the body, your body goes out of balance and your immune system is weakened. When this occurs your body can not fight off any of the viruses or bacteria that you pick up, thus you get sick more often, with more severity, and for longer periods of time. You also have an environment that is very likely to produce illness and disease. I pointed out earlier that the number one cause of the high amounts of toxicity in the body is prescription and nonprescription drugs. The amount of sickness, the increased severity and increased duration, is in direct relation to the increase in prescription and non-prescription drug use.

However, illness and disease become complicated issues when you look at the hundreds of variables that are involved. I want to generally address what you should do, and then in the next chapter I'll give you some specifics depending on your current situation (keeping in mind that I am not a medical doctor). I am not giving medical advice, and I can not cure any disease. As a matter of fact I believe that there is not a single person or substance on the planet that can cure a disease in the traditional, medically accepted sense . The only thing that happens is a healthcare practitioner can do some things, using all-natural remedies, that will help your body heal itself. No one can "cure" a disease. Only your body can cure or heal itself. I do believe that there are certain things you can do to help your body heal itself better, or cure itself of illness, sickness and disease. I do believe that there are certain things you can do that can temporarily address some of the symptoms, ultimately allowing your body to regain its natural balanced state where illness and disease can not exist.

So let me expand on this point. The "too much toxins in the body" comes down to this:

1. What goes in the body
2. What comes out of the body
3. Exercise
4. Rest
5. Thoughts
6. What you say

So let's go through the list and address some common misconceptions, and see what you should be doing if you want to virtually eliminate any disease. Maybe some of you reading this book have a disease or know someone who does. Maybe others are concerned about getting a disease and your major interest is doing the steps necessary to prevent that disease or illness or sickness. Keep in mind the natural state of the human body is vibrant health. If you have any type of discomfort, illness, disease or sickness you are out of balance. It is not the natural state that your body was designed for. Your body was designed to be healthy and never get sick. Think about that.

The six areas listed above have a direct relation to toxicity in the body. It is interesting to note that when you are toxic, your body becomes highly acidic. Your body pH should be alkaline. When your body pH is acidic you are susceptible to illness and disease. When your body pH is alkaline, you virtually can never get sick! Every single person who has cancer has a pH that is too acidic! Let me show you how each of the above six areas cause you to become too toxic, thus more acidic, and thus more prone to illness and disease.

Let's look at what we put in our body. As I mentioned, we put things in our body through our mouth, through our nose, through our eyes, through our ears, and through our skin. Let's talk about what goes in through our mouth.

I think Jack LaLane said it best. Jack LaLane is an incredible human being. He is in his nineties; he is vibrant, healthy and strong. He doesn't get sick. He is a dynamic, healthy individual. Jack says: "If man made it, don't eat it." That's basically the bottom line. What you put in your mouth should be 100 percent natural. If man made it, you shouldn't eat it. Now, if you go out and eat an apple you may think, "Ah, this is an apple; man didn't make it, therefore I can eat it." Well, we have a problem. Virtually all fruits and vegetables are, in today's day and age, man-made.

Did you know that virtually all fruits and vegetables have been genetically modified by man to become more disease resistant? You have to understand that the food industry is just the same as the pharmaceutical industry—it's all about the money.

A food manufacturer, or for that matter a farmer, is in business and has to sell more of his product and produce that product at a lower cost to make more money. So what farmers do is say, "Hmm, how can I grow the most apples or the most carrots or the most onions out of my field? How can I produce them in the shortest period of time, at the lowest cost, so I can sell them at the highest possible profit?" The answer is: Mess around with mother nature and change these natural fruits and vegetables with some man-made concoction that came out of a laboratory so that they grow bigger and faster totally against the natural course of things, and are resistant to disease. "That way I can make sure I have a full crop and I can sell more of my produce and make more money." So through genetic modification, your all-natural carrot is no longer all-natural, it is really a man-made product.

But it gets worse, because that farmer has to squeeze in and produce more carrots per acre in order to make more profit. He uses chemical fertilizers and chemical pesticides and herbicides that he sprays on these natural products like carrots. When you then take that natural piece of fruit or vegetable, it is loaded with toxic chemicals. It also has much less nutritional value than it would have fifty or sixty years ago. It has been said that you would need to eat up to five times the amount of food your grandparents did just to receive the same nutritional value. That's why if you are going to eat fruits and vegetables—or any food for that matter—which I highly encourage of course, they must be organically grown. Grains such as rice and wheat are the same. You need to be buying organically grown food.

In America, as opposed to many other countries, virtually everything you put in your mouth is toxic or contains toxins. Virtually everything made by man is toxic. This does not mean everything that is natural is not toxic. There are plants that are poisonous and if consumed could kill you. But, virtually everything made by man is a poison. Today, we put more toxins in our body than ever before.

Virtually everything that you put in your mouth has pesticides, herbicides, antibiotics, growth hormone, genetically altered material, or chemical food additives. Even when you eat an apple you are taking in all the deadly chemicals that were used in the growing and harvesting of that apple. All of our fruits, vegetables, grains, nuts and seeds are grown with highly poisonous chemical fertilizers, pesticides and herbicides. Many have been genetically modified, turning them into poisonous material. Even when you consume fresh fruits and vegetables, you are ingesting small amounts of poison.

The same conditions apply in the meat industry. Like farmers and other food producers, the meat industry needs to create a lot of product cheaply and quickly, and sell it for as high a profit as possible. To that end, the industry uses growth hormones to speed an animal's growth (contributing to the record levels of obesity and early puberty in our children); antibiotics to keep the animal healthy in unsanitary and inhumane, though economical, conditions (explaining the contemporary failure of antibiotics—the wonder drug of the 20th century—in humans);

feeds the animals unnatural feed diets that not only pump more chemicals into the meat, but also so upset the animals' systems that they become out of balance and pass that imbalance along to those who consume the meat. Many meat products are also "aged." This means the dead animal flesh is allowed to rot, permitting deadly bacteria to grow. Remember, if it's not organic, if man has made it, don't eat it!

The same holds true with dairy products. Because of the use of drugs, growth hormones, pasteurization and homogenization, dairy products today are a major health concern unless they are organic, not pasteurized, and not homogenized. There are two other things to consider when looking at dairy products, one of which is pasteurization and the other homogenization. Pasteurization simply heats the dairy product to a very high temperature to kill any bacteria. The major problem is it also kills the living enzymes that are in the milk, making it much harder to digest in the body and thus making the milk a totally unnatural product. But more importantly, and more dangerous, is homogenization.

Do you remember the milkman? We used to have the milkman come to the house to deliver milk. Why did we have to have a milkman? Why couldn't we just buy our milk in the store? The reason is the milk went bad very quickly. It spoiled within just a few days.

The food industry said "We're losing money by not selling milk in our stores. We can't sell milk because it goes bad too quickly." So the industry came up with an incredible solution, a process called homogenization. When the milkman delivered our milk, you may remember that the cream separated from the milk. You had to shake up the milk before you drank it. The process of homogenization actually spins the milk at a very high rate breaking down the clusters of molecules within the milk so that you don't have any separation of the cream and the milk. Therefore the milk will not spoil within a few days, it can actually last a few weeks before going bad. Now that the food industry can have milk shipped to them, they can put it on the store shelf and they can sell it, there is no more need for the milkman. The problem is homogenized and pasteurized milk, and all dairy products, are unnatural. The clusters of molecules are so small that when you ingest them they virtually scar your arteries. They clog up your digestive system, making it very difficult to digest food, which is one of the major caus-es of acid reflux disease, obesity, and constipation. And the scarring of the arteries causes the LDL cholesterol to attach itself to the artery, which is one of the major causes or arteriosclerosis, which is one of the major causes of heart disease. The bottom line is pasteurized and homogenized dairy products are unnatural, raw dairy products are nat-ural. Organic, raw, natural dairy products are natural. Remember Jack LaLane said, "If man made it, don't eat it."

When you eat fish you are only slightly better off. Many kinds of fish are "farmed," meaning that highly toxic feed and chemicals are used to make the fish grow unnaturally fast to unnaturally large sizes. Other poisonous chemicals are used in the processing of the fish before sale to consumers. When you consume this "man-made" fish, you are also taking in all the poisons and toxins that have been used in its produc-tion. Fish in the wild are much better. However, because of the massive dumping of poisonous chemicals into out lakes, rivers, and oceans, many wild fish have been found to have abnormally high levels of toxic chemicals in them. When you eat ANY food that has been produced by a food manufacturer, the fact is that you are 100 percent guaranteed to be ingesting highly toxic and poisonous man-made chemicals.

What else do we put in our body through our mouth? If it's in a box, if it's in a jar, if it's in a can, it's been processed by the food industry. Keep in mind that the food industry consists of publicly traded corpo-rations that have one objective: to make more money and increase shareholder value. And the way they do that is to sell more food, and produce that food at a lower cost. Always remember that, it's always about the money.

The food industry puts tens of thousands of chemical ingredients into the food and, in many cases, they do not have to list those ingre-dients on the label. How do they get away with that? Through our lob-byist friends, and by paying off politicians and members of the Food and Drug Administration. It's all about the money.

So why is that bad?

The additives being put in the food are unnatural, toxic chemicals. They adversely affect the body; they suppress your immune system making it more susceptible to disease; they make you age quicker, and they turn your body from the natural alkaline pH state to the acid pH state, which means you can easily be prone to cancer, heart disease, diabetes, allergies, etc., etc., etc.

Not only are these chemical additives toxic, when they are put into the food the processing of the food strips away much of the nutritional value. As I mentioned before, if you were to eat a regular apple, it would have only one-fifth of the nutrition of an apple fifty years ago. But once the food is processed and put in a box or a can, you're going to have to eat 100 times more to get the same nutritional value; nutrition is virtually wiped out. So in addition to having the poisons put in your system from the chemicals not even listed on the label, the food you are getting has almost no nutritional value. Plus, these food additives actually block absorption of nutrients. Not only are you not getting enough nutrients from the food you are eating, but what little nutrients you are getting are being blocked and not absorbed. This means everyone has nutritional deficiencies causing imbalance, and a weakened immune system, which makes you both susceptible to viruses and bacteria, and causes your body to develop diseases and pain.

Why are these food additives put in the food anyway? Well it's very interesting. I was actually at a health spa where there was a gentleman who was a senior executive at a major food processing company, one of the largest producers of canned goods in the world. We were talking about the food additives and, yes, he admitted that there are thousands and thousands of chemical additives put into the food, and many of these additives are not listed on the label at all. I suggested that these food additives were dangerous to a person's health and were one of the reasons why people are so sick today. He assured me that these chemicals were totally safe, and that they were in such small amounts that they would have no effect whatsoever on the human body.

I then asked him a question. I said that, if they are totally safe, if I were to give you a glass of one of these chemicals, would you drink it? He stammered and stuttered and went back and forth a few times. I must have asked him the question ten times without getting an answer.

Finally he said no, he wouldn't drink it because it could potentially be a problem. He finally admitted that the ingredients were, in fact, toxic. But, he repeated that, because they were in such small amounts, they had no effect at all on the human body. I then asked him the million dollar question. I said, "If you are putting such a small amount in, and these ingredients have no effect at all on the human body, then they must have no effect at all on the food. So why do you have to put them in the food?" Again, he couldn't answer the question. After grilling this man, he finally admitted that they in fact have a **major** effect. They preserve the food and give it taste. But I could tell that there was something else that these ingredients did that he wasn't telling. I then searched through my network of insiders, my network of whistleblowers, and here is what I discovered:

The food industry, just like the tobacco industry is hiding a dirty little secret. The food industry is putting ingredients in the food knowingly and on purpose, because these ingredients make a person hungry, make a person fat and make them addicted to the food. Now listen and pay attention, because what I am telling you is one of the biggest news stories of the century! The food industry, an industry of publicly traded companies, is all about the money.

Imagine this conversation actually happening: A junior executive walks into the boardroom and says "Gentlemen, in order for us to increase shareholder value and the price of our stock, we need to sell more food and produce this food at the lowest possible cost. And I have the solution. There are certain ingredients that, when mixed together and added to the food, actually make people hungrier. So that when they buy our product, they actually have to eat more of it, they can't stop eating it, it makes them hungrier. There are also certain chemicals we can put in the food that will actually make a person get fatter even if they don't eat that much; and the fatter they get, the hungrier they'll get, and they will have to consume more food and they will have to buy more food. And there are certain ingredients that we can put in the food that gets the people chemically addicted to the food, so that they have to have the food, they can't stop eating it; and if they stop eating it, they will get headaches, nauseous, they'll be upset, depressed and anxious until they eat some of the food, very similar to opium or cocaine."

Is this crazy? Well, remember Coca Cola? Coca Cola was colored sweetened water which had cocaine in it. Coca Cola was the name because Coca referred to the coca plant and Cola referred to the cola nut. The cola nut had the caffeine, and the coca or the cocaine got the person physically addicted. It was quietly removed back in the 1920s, without much fanfare or media exposure.

Right now as you are reading this, the food industry—like every other industry—has to increase profits, and the only way they can do so is to sell you more food. Why is it that Americans are the fattest people on the planet? Remember, it's all about the money.

Oh, there are a couple of other scary things as well. Many of the ingredients they put in the food make you depressed, which is really good for the drug companies because if you are depressed, you have to go to the drug companies to handle your depression. Interestingly enough, some of the food additives which are put in the food to make you depressed are manufactured by the same companies that sell you the antidepressant drugs. It's a fantastic money-making business folks. Remember, it's all about the money.

There is another reason why these chemical additives are bad. As I mentioned, when we consume food we are getting certain nutrients. When chemicals are put into the food, the processing of the food strips away much of the nutritional value in the food. If you were to eat a regular apple, you would have to eat five times as many apples to match the nutrients in one apple fifty years ago. But once the food is processed and put in a box or a can, you're going to have to eat 100 times to get the same nutritional value. So in addition to having the poisons put in your system from the chemicals which aren't even listed on the label, the food you are getting has almost no nutritional value. Plus, these food additives block the absorption of nutrients. Not only are you not getting enough nutrients from the food you are eating, but what little nutrients you are getting are being blocked and not absorbed. This means everyone has nutritional deficiencies causing imbalance, and a weakened immune system making you both susceptible to viruses and bacteria and causing your body to develop diseases and pain. But there is another problem. The energy that you get from food is virtually wiped out.

Without giving a physics lesson, when you eat anything you are getting the energy from that thing. How do we know this is true? Well, think about it. You take a pot and you put soil in it. You put in ten pounds of soil, and you put in one little tiny seed, and every day you add some water, and at the end of a year you have this big plant. Well, take the plant out, shake off the soil from the roots and weigh the soil. Guess what? You still have ten pounds of soil. The only thing you added was some water. If you were to measure the water, you may have added about five pounds of water. Theoretically, the plant should weigh no more than five pounds if it grabbed 100 percent of the water. But the plant weighs fifty pounds. Wow! What happened? How did fifty pounds of mass and matter magically appear? It didn't eat the soil, the ten pounds of soil is still there, and there were only five pounds of water added. How did that magically generate out of nothing?

Human beings are the same. If you take a little baby, and you weigh every bit of food that goes in and then subtract all the excretions that come out through the urine, the stool, and sweating through the skin, you would see that whatever goes in comes out. If tens pounds of food and water are put in, guess what? Ten pounds of stuff comes out, but the little baby grows from fifteen pounds to fifty pounds to 150 pounds. But everything that goes in, all the liquid and everything we eat, comes out. How does that happen? Well guess what? Science really can't give you an answer. The answer is that we get the energy from the food and the sunlight and the air, and that's how matter is manifested—it's the energy.

So if we go through everything that we put in our mouth, whatever we eat and whatever we drink, ask yourself: is it natural, or has it been screwed up by some greedy individual who doesn't care about your health, who doesn't care if you get sick, who doesn't care if you're depressed, or if you get fat? The only thing they care about is making money. Remember, it's always all about the money.

So what do we eat and drink? Well, ideally you want to eat all-natural things, fruits and vegetables, and get them organic. When you cook them it destroys some of the living enzymes, so raw is better than cooked. Should you become a vegetarian? I don't know if you should be a vegetarian or not. Everyone is a little different. What works for one person may work slightly better or worse for someone else. I can tell you this. I believe that if you add or increase the amount of raw fruits and vegetables in your diet, you'll be better off.

Here's the other big problem. You can't look at food labels, you have to read the ingredients. Because if the label says all-natural, it's usually a big lie. Why? The food industry has lobbied the politicians to allow certain totally man-made ingredients to be classified as all-natural. Keep in mind that there are over 10,000 ingredients that don't even have to be put on the label. So if you see something that says "all-natural," it just means that the government has allowed them to put that on so they can sell more of the food. Ideally, if it's in a box or can, don't even eat it. Some people go into "health food stores" and assume that everything that is in the health food store is good for them. It's not, you have to read labels; and ideally, if it's in a box, if it's in a bottle or jar, don't consume it.

Which leads me to restaurants. The big question is: What can I eat in restaurants? The answer: nothing!

You may say, "Well, I can't live like that." I know it is unrealistic for you to completely change what you have been doing your whole life. But realistically, there is nothing in a restaurant that can be classified as safe. Yes, I eat at restaurants. Why? Because I'm not fanatical, and I am not asking you to be fanatical. Now I do know some people who are fanatical. They eat nothing but raw organic food, and these people are absolutely amazing physical specimens. However, I live in the real world, and so do you. Just do the best you can. Realistically, stay away from anything in the fast food restaurant. They are categorically the worst.

Let me say this again because it is so important. There are over 15,000 toxic chemicals that are allowed to be added to food without being listed on the label. Every year, the food industry puts a higher percentage of toxic chemicals in our food. These chemicals are produced in secret laboratories where the security is higher than Fort Knox! When asked why these chemicals are put into the food, the answers are vague and ambiguous. However, from information I have received from "insiders," I can now blow the whistle on the real reasons these chemicals are being added to our food without our knowledge. Remember, it always goes back to "it's all about the money."

Food companies have one goal: to make more money. The only way they can make more money is to produce the food the cheapest way possible, sell it at the highest price possible, and sell more and more food. The scientists who work in these secret laboratories are developing chemicals and combinations of chemicals that are added to our food and not put on the label. This is legal because the food industry, through the lobbyists' system of legal bribery, has gotten Congress to pass certain legislation allowing this to occur. These secret poisonous chemicals are specifically designed to do the following things:

- **Preserve the food.** In order to produce food as cheaply as possible, it is sometimes required that chemicals be added to the food so that it will not spoil even after years of just sitting around. We have all heard the story of the thirty-year-old Twinkie that looked and tasted the same as it did the day it was manufactured.

- **Taste and texture.** Much of today's food is produced in such an unnatural way that is has very little nutritional value and very little taste. Chemicals must be added to make the food taste like it is supposed to taste. A major hamburger chain adds a chemical to its hamburgers to make them taste like a hamburger!

- **To make you hungry!** You are reading this right. The food industry knows that it must sell MORE food to make more money. If it can add a chemical that actually makes you hungrier, you will eat more food and they will make more money!

- **To make you fatter.** Fat people eat more food. Chemicals are being added to our food that actually make us gain weight. The more fat people there are, the more profits there are for the food industry. The most shocking part of this is one such chemical put in most "diet food." How sad that an unknowing consumer buys some food that has the word "diet" on it in the hopes of losing some weight, when actually eating the food causes them to **gain weight**.

- **To get the person addicted to the product!** Food manufacturers are knowingly putting chemicals into the food that cause the consumer to become physically addicted to it. We know that drugs, which are simply chemicals, can be incredibly physically and emotionally addictive. This practice is not new. In the book *The Real Thing: The Truth and Power at the Coca Cola Company,* the story of how cocaine was an important ingredient in Coca-Cola is exposed. One of the main reasons cocaine was such an important ingredient was that the consumer unknowingly became addicted to Coca-Cola. Having a person addicted to your product is good for your profits, but bad for the poor bastard who is addicted.

- **To give you disease.** As outrageous as it seems, it appears that insiders know that certain "food additives" cause specific diseases. If you knew that huge numbers of people would be coming down with a certain disease in the next five or ten years, you could invest in drug companies that are producing drugs that will be prescribed for this "new disease." When I talk about the greed of the people involved, 99 percent of the people have no comprehension of just how the love of money has taken almost absolute control over these people's actions, ethics, and morals. Think about Howard Hughes. He was one of the richest men in the world, if not the richest. Yet, on his death bed, up until the hour he died, he was still trying to make more money!

Obviously, what I am saying here is my opinion and my conclusions. It is vehemently denied by the food industry and the FDA, but think about the same type of denials for years by the tobacco industry. I believe time will prove me absolutely correct.

The other important issue relating to the amounts of these chemicals is that chemicals ingested in the body do not necessarily leave the body. It appears that chemical fertilizers, pesticides, herbicides, growth hormone, nonprescription and prescription drugs, and food additives such as artificial sweeteners, stay in the body and lodge in the fatty tissues. Since our brain is mostly fat, a large percentage of these chemicals accumulate there over the years. This is believed to be one of the main reasons that there is such a massive increase in depression, stress and anxiety, and learning disabilities like attention deficit disorder.

When we eat this our body gets "stressed." Anything we put in our body that stresses our body does two things:

1. It suppresses your immune system, making you more susceptible to disease.

2. It can turn your body from the natural alkaline pH state, in which disease and illness and sickness can not survive, to an acidic state in which diseases like cancer, heart disease and diabetes can thrive.

You have to ask yourself a question when you put something in your mouth: Could this have been made 100 years ago? If it couldn't, don't eat it. The reason it is being processed the way it is, is because somebody is making money. Remember, it's always about the money.

You see, the food industry is very, very persuasive. They try to make you believe that science is better than nature. Science is not better than nature. Science is only better for the food manufacturer, because it allows him to make more money. A good example of this is margarine. Margarine is produced by hydrogenating oil. What does that mean? It means taking oil and spinning it until it becomes a solid. The problem with hydrogenated oil is that it scars the arteries and causes heart disease. It's classified now as a trans fat, and finally we are hearing a little bit about the dangers of trans fats. We are finally being told that, oops! we've been saying to you that margarine is much better for you than butter; I guess we were wrong. I guess the man-made product is doing all types of damage to your health and we just didn't know about it. Or maybe they did know about it but, were making too much money and just decided not tell anybody.

We have all-natural sugar, and then we have artificial sweeteners like saccharine and aspartame. You are led to believe that the chemical man-made sweeteners are so much better for your health than all-natural sugar. Nothing could be further from the truth. The artificial sweeteners are one of the major reasons that you are fat. They also cause depression. There was a great book written about this, *Exitotoxins—The Taste That Kills,* and another one called *Aspartame (NutraSweet®)—Is It Safe?* If it's made by man, don't eat it! Don't be tricked by all the advertising. Remember, it's all about the money.

The food industry has to convince you that you have to buy their chemically produced, man-made food stuffs, and that it's better than something all-natural. It's a lie! They are only trying to persuade you so they can make more money.

The processing of food causes another problem. Certain processing techniques change a natural food into an unnatural toxin. Let's go back to the dairy industry. How would you define milk? We hear a lot about milk. The dairy association obviously wants you to drink more milk. Remember, they don't care about you, they only care about the profits of its members that it represents, which in this case is all the people in the dairy industry. There have been thousands of studies on milk. Some say milk is good, others say milk is bad. Is there only one kind of milk? What kind of milk was used in the studies? If I were to tell you "milk" is good for you, do you think milk is milk is milk? There are many definitions and many kinds of milk. For example:

Is it cow's milk or goat's milk? Is the animal giving the milk injected with growth hormone and antibiotics? Is the animal giving the milk eating a natural diet of grass, or a man-made diet of genetically altered corn, ground up dead animals and other chemically produced material designed to increase milk production? Is the cow giving the milk allowed to wander and walk in the way nature intended, or is the animal confined to a pen and not allowed to move for its entire life? Has the animal been genetically modified and bred specifically for increased milk production and profits, or is it a natural animal bred according to nature? Is the animal sick and diseased, or healthy? Is the animal milked by a machine, causing blood and pus to be in the milk, or milked in a natural way without blood and pus? Is the milk heated to 220 degrees for thirty minutes, killing off all the natural living enzymes (pasteurization), or is the milk immediately put into cold storage? Is the milk immediately put in a glass bottle and delivered to your door by the milkman within four hours after coming out of the animal, or is the milk processed by adding chemicals to it, which are not listed on the label, and homogenized?

You see, if I say cow's milk or goat's milk is good for you, I mean the all-natural, organic non-man-made version. Once the food industry gets involved and starts messing around so that they can make more money, everything gets screwed up and the new man-made unnatural products become toxic to the body. If it's made by man, don't eat it. Remember, science is not better than nature except when it comes to making money.

Another common food processing technique is *irradiation*. This is when foods such as fruits, vegetables, grains, meat, poultry and fish are zapped with radioactive beams of energy designed to kill any harmful bacteria, so you won't get violently sick or die when you eat it. This has been needed because the food processing system is producing food that has a higher chance of having deadly pathogens, therefore causing sickness or death. Irradiation changes the energetic frequency of the food, giving the food a frequency that is no longer life sustaining, but rather toxic to the body. This has been shown with Kirlian photography. If you take an apple and take a picture of it with Kirlian photography, you see a very beautiful pattern of energy surrounding the apple. If the apple is zapped with a microwave and a second Kirlian photograph is taken, you see the energy pattern around the apple has radically changed. The pattern is now jagged, rough, and erratic. The energy pattern is more like arsenic, a deadly poison. So, the processing of food changes food from a healthy, natural, life-sustaining fuel, to an unnatural man-made toxic poison.

If you read the labels of everything you put in your mouth, you would see the name of various chemicals. All the chemicals listed are dangerous man-made chemicals. They are poisons. If you were to take any of those chemicals and ingest a large amount at one time, you would probably die. Therefore they are in fact poisons. Think about the 15,000 chemicals that are in our food that do not have to be listed on the label.

• • •

Now let's talk about what else you put in your mouth, primarily what you drink. There are two problems here. The first one is most people don't drink enough water, and the second one is the water you drink is incredibly toxic. All tap water has chemicals put in it, primarily chlorine and fluoride. The level of toxicity of both chlorine and fluoride is incredible. Drinking chlorinated water, which is virtually all tap water, causes scarring of the arteries. When the arteries are scarred, the LDL cholesterol attaches itself to the artery causing arteriosclerosis.

Most people are dehydrated, which causes all types of medical problems including pain, stiffness, arthritis, asthma, allergies and other medical issues. Dehydration means the cells just simply don't have enough fluid. It can affect your energy and your sleep, but the major thing that it has an effect on is the ability to get toxins and waste matter out of the body and out of cells. Cells can live forever in a laboratory, so long as the fluid in which the cell is living is constantly cleaned and changed. If you take a cell and basically put in fluid, the cell excretes waste matter and toxins. As long as you clean that environment and get rid of the waste matter and toxins, the cell never seems to age, and that's pretty staggering! That's why cleansing and getting the toxins out of your system is so important. It's also why putting the least amount of toxins in your body is so important.

The debate is on about the best type of water. The basic types of water you have in your environment are tap water, purified water, spring water and distilled water.

Tap water is absolutely the worst kind of water in the world because virtually all tap water is contaminated. All tap water has chlorine in it, and most tap water has fluoride in it. Fluoride is one of the most toxic chemicals in the world. It is a product that comes from the manufacture of superphosphic fertilizers, and is so toxic it can't be dumped anywhere. Through lobbying, fluoride was then sold to municipalities and dumped in our water supplies under the disguise of being good for our teeth. It's a big lie and nothing could be further from the truth. Fluoride is toxic and dangerous, and should not be consumed. Fluoride adversely affects virtually every organ in the body, primarily your thyroid gland. It can be seen that the areas in America that have the most fluoride in the water have the highest obesity rates because people's metabolisms go down. Fluoride makes you depressed and causes all types of physical problems.

Certainly spring water is better than tap water. But certain agencies and interest groups publish misleading stories about bottled water not being any better than tap water because the bacteria count in bottled water is higher than that in tap water. These stories point out that there is no bacteria in tap water because of the chlorine. The problem is, chlorine kills living organisms. We too are living organisms. Chlorine is a poison, and it is put into the water supply to kill living organisms. When we drink it, we're drinking poison. Yes, we are taking it in small amounts, but it's still a highly poisonous chemical and should not be consumed. There is nothing wrong with bacteria. We get exposed to bacteria every single day. That's how our immune systems get strengthened, that's how we live. Our body is exposed to bacteria and germs and viruses and we have natural immunities to those things. The more we are exposed to them the better off our systems are.

What kind of water do I drink? I have a reverse osmosis unit in my house. I have the water in my entire house filtered. I also have a distiller which, in addition to steam distillation, also gets rid of the energetic memory attached to the water. I do drink bottled water when I travel. I do not drink bottled water that is filtered or purified. I drink bottled spring water.

Let me digress here for a moment. People are always talking about cholesterol, cholesterol, cholesterol. It's a great business for the drug companies. They get you to believe you need to lower your cholesterol. But cholesterol is not the cause of heart disease. There are people with 600 cholesterol counts that have absolutely no arteriosclerosis, no blockages and no heart disease. And there are people with cholesterol counts of 100 who have massive blockages and are dropping dead from heart attacks and need triple bypass surgeries. The amount of cholesterol in your blood is not the problem. The problem only occurs when the cholesterol attaches itself to the artery, thus clogging the artery and restricting the blood flow. When it's restricted you need bypass surgery, thus says the medical community. There are all-natural alternatives to bypass surgery as well. Which are more effective, get to the root cause instead of just handling the symptom. The question, however, really is not how much cholesterol you have, but what causes the cholesterol to attach itself to the artery? The cholesterol will only attach itself to the artery when the artery is damaged. If the artery is not damaged the cholesterol just goes through the blood without any problem whatsoever, and you will never have heart disease no matter what your cholesterol count is. So the question is, what causes damage to the artery?

Primarily, there are three things that cause the artery to get scarred. And its when the artery is scarred that the cholesterol begins the attaching process, and that's when and how you get arteriosclerosis and heart disease.

1. **Chlorinated water**. Chlorine in the water that you drink and shower and bathe in or swim in causes massive scarring of the arteries, which in turn means, no matter how much cholesterol you have or don't have, whatever cholesterol is there will attach itself and begin the clogging process.

2. **Hydrogenated oils or trans fats**. As you look at virtually 90 percent of the food produced in boxes, if you were to actually read the label you'd see the words "hydrogenated oil" or "partially hydrogenated oil." These are trans fats. Margarine, for example, is hydrogenated oil. These trans fats scar the arteries, causing heart disease and arteriosclerosis.

3. **Homogenized dairy products**. People say, "Well I drink low fat milk or low fat yogurt." The fat has nothing to do with it. You are being scammed, you are being lied to, you are being misled. It's not the fat that is the problem. Keep in mind that when they make a low fat product, it's not a natural product, it's man-made. What's unnatural is the homogenization process. The homogenization process in either the milk or the cheese, when you consume a dairy product that has been homogenized, will cause the arteries to get scarred. These are the three major causes of arteriosclerosis.

The bottom line is no matter what they are called, there are in fact more toxic chemicals in our water and food supply than ever before in history. These poisons are getting into our bodies primarily by:

• Drinking the water

• Eating or drinking anything made with water

- Eating any food that was grown with the water
- Eating any meat, poultry, fish or dairy where the animal drank water
- Showering, bathing or swimming in water

Since our skin is the largest organ in the body, it has been reported that we absorb more toxins by taking one shower than by drinking five glasses of water. In a shower, not only is the water with all the toxins being absorbed through the skin, many of the most volatile and dangerous toxins are turned into a gas created by the steam. These toxic fumes in your shower are then inhaled. A shower is practically a gas chamber filled with poisonous gas chemicals. Steam rooms, hot tubs and swimming pools are places where you will absorb the highest levels of toxins. The paradox is we think of these particular areas as being the healthiest.

The poisoned water supply is another significant factor relating to how toxins get into our body. By now it won't surprise you to learn how we are being misled by the news media and government agencies about the purity and safety of our water supply. Remember that chlorine and fluoride are the two main poisons that are in our water supply and are the reason our water is so unhealthy. Yet, the government and news media rates the quality of our water based on the amount of chlorine and fluoride in it! The more chlorine and fluoride in the water the healthier it is, claims the government! They even say that tap water is better than spring water because tap water has chlorine and fluoride in it and spring water does not. This is yet another way you are being lied to, deceived and brainwashed into thinking that chemicals are better than something in a natural state.

Let's talk about other things you put in through your mouth that you drink: coffee, tea, sodas, and alcohol. Remember the rule: If it's man made, don't put it in your body.

What about coffee? Well let's start with pure, clean water—not tap water. Let's take a coffee been that has been organically grown and simply ground up. If it's organic there are no chemicals, no herbicides, no pesticides and no chemicals used in the processing. It seems pretty reasonable in moderation. It appears to be okay. Teas are the same, real organic tea. I'm talking tea leaves, not tea bags, which tea drinkers will say is nothing but flavored water when you make it.

What about carbonated sodas? I very rarely, if ever, drink them. I would never in a million years drink a diet soda because the chemical sweeteners, in my opinion, are some of the most toxic things you could put in your body. On occasion I will drink a Coca Cola from a bottle, not a can. The problem, however, with virtually all carbonated beverages is they block calcium absorption. Calcium is one of the most important building blocks of nutrition.

What about alcohol? If you come to my house I have an array of liqueurs, spirits, wine and beer primarily for guests. What's the ideal scene? Drink water and nothing else. Tea can be very therapeutic, as well as wine. Try to drink mostly pure water, then some tea, then wine, then other alcohol and everything else rarely if ever.

Ah! What about juices? If man made it, don't put it in your body. I would never buy juice out of a can or bottle and drink it. Why? If you've ever gone to see how these products are made, you would see why. People think juice is juice is juice. It's simply not true! I happen to have a juice machine in my house. I also have in my back yard some fruit trees. So when I want some juice, I usually walk out, pick some oranges or grapefruits, walk in, peel them and juice them. And I get delicious, organic, pure juice.

Well how is that different from juice you buy at the store? A couple of major differences:

Remember, it's all about the money. The people who sell these products are trying to sell more product at a lower cost. How do they do that? Well, first and foremost let's take orange juice. What will happen is they'll find the worst oranges in the world that they couldn't sell, and that's what they make their juice from. Keep in mind that these oranges have been produced in the "conventional" way, with chemical fertilizers, pesticides, herbicides and genetic engineering. That's conventional? No! That's weird, that's bizarre, that's wrong!

They then pick the fruit that can't be sold, and that's what they make the juice from. The problem is that in the processing of the juice in the plants, bacteria and mold can easily develop, contaminating the product. So by law the product has to be pasteurized, which means the product has to be heated to 220 degrees for thirty minutes to kill any amount of bacteria so you don't get sick as you drink it. This kills all the living natural enzymes and destroys the natural energy surrounding that natural fruit. It is then filtered, and in many cases sugar, which is not listed on the label, is added to make the product sweeter. If sugar is not added, the filtering process and the pasteurization process make the product much sweeter. So you are getting a product that is much, much sweeter than in nature. The best example of this is filtered apple juice. When you look at apple juice that is super clear, it is so much sweeter than natural apple juice that I make at my house on my juicing machine. It has no living enzymes, and it's virtually a massive sugar high. It's just a man-made product under the disguise of a natural, healthy product. It's not healthy; it's man made, it's tainted with chemicals and toxins, and because of the processing is just not healthy. Juice is good, but only if you make it in your home with organic fruits and vegetables, and drink your juice right away. Once you have juiced the product and air gets to it, it begins to oxidize and lose its nutritional value. So if you have a juice machine in your house, you get organic fruits and vegetables, you make juice and you drink it.

But why should you drink juice anyway? That's not natural; 100 years ago we didn't have juice machines. That's a very, very good question. The answer is this: Even if you buy organic fruits and vegetables today, because over the years the soil has been depleted of much of its nutritional value and energy, today's fruits and vegetables don't have the energy or the nutritional value that they did 100 years ago. Even organic fruits and vegetables have less than they did 100 years ago. So a good alternative is to juice them. The nutritional value and the life force energy is in the juice. The fiber in the fruits and vegetables is still needed for other bodily functions such as the elimination through the colon, so you still need to eat the whole fruit and vegetable. But you can get the nutritional value through the juice. It is much better than taking vitamin and mineral tablets if you're going to juice.

So to summarize: If it's made by man, don't put it in your body.

How toxins get in your body through your skin

The skin is the largest organ in the body. Anything put on the skin is absorbed and gets into the body. Even science admits this to be true.

Drugs are administered topically on the skin. These drugs wind up in the bloodstream within minutes. Everything you put on your skin gets into your bloodstream. Our friends at the FDA have determined that many chemicals are for external use only. They are poisonous and can not be taken internally because they can kill you. But remember, whatever you put on your skin winds up in your body. Do you understand the problem here? We put things on our skin such as lotions, moisturizers, sun screens, cosmetics, soap, shampoo etc. Virtually every one of these things contains ingredients that even the FDA says are so poisonous and so deadly that they can not be taken internally. Yet, they are allowed to be put on your skin. The FDA knows that these poisons get into your body via the skin, yet because of the tremendous pressure by lobbyists and politicians, the manufacturers are allowed to put these dangerous ingredients in their products. A Swiss study concluded that five of the most common ingredients in sun screens cause cancer. It is no wonder why the more sun screen you use, the higher the chance that you will get skin cancer. The sun does not cause skin cancer, the sun screens do! Underarm deodorants and antiperspirants contain deadly chemicals that many people believe to be a major cause of breast cancer in women.

If you can't eat it, do not put it on your skin!

We absorb many toxins through our nose

These are primarily the poisons that are in the air. Where you live and work determines the amount of pollutants in the air. Most major cities contend that the air is filled with poisonous chemicals. We breathe every second, therefore we are absorbing toxins every second. However, there are many toxins in the air that most people are not aware of. Air fresheners are one of the worst. Talk about misleading advertising, how in the world can they claim that these products "freshen" the air? These products contain deadly, poisonous chemicals. Would you consider opening the can and drinking the air freshener? Read the label, they even tell you how poisonous the ingredients are! These products eliminate odors by having you spray a deadly poison in the air. This poison kills all of the receptors in the nose so that you can not smell the offending odor any more. They don't eliminate odors, they eliminate your ability to smell them!

Other toxins include mold, dust, pollens, and the fumes emitted from carpeting, glue, paint, mattresses, the soaps used in the cleaning of sheets and clothing, and air conditioning units. Think about the term "air conditioning." How can putting chemicals in the air be called "conditioning" the air? Air conditioning units cool the air, but load the air with contaminants. The most important nutrient to the body is oxygen. A man can live for weeks without food, days without water, but only a few minutes without air. Any aroma that you smell means something is going into your body. Even if you lived on a farm, the smell of manure means particles of manure are entering your body.

In today's world, the fact is that we are inhaling toxins on a regular basis. It is virtually impossible to eliminate them. However, it is entirely possible to dramatically reduce the amount of toxins you are inhaling. It's also interesting to note that what you inhale has a very immediate and profound effect on such things as appetite, digestion, moods, depression, anxiety, irritability, and sleep. Reducing the toxins that you breathe can have a very profound and dramatic impact on your health.

The eyes

Toxins get in through the eyes in a similar fashion to the skin. The eyes also, in addition to the skin, are the entry point of solar energy from the sun. The sun is not a toxin, as you are being led to believe. The lack of sun causes deficiencies in the body, leading to imbalances and disease. The major form of toxins that come in through the eyes is images that cause bad emotions. Today there are more violent images on television, in the movies, in newspapers and magazines, video games, and books than ever before. Repeated exposure to negative, ugly, disturbing images causes the body to become acidic. Today, people are being exposed to over one thousand times the amount of negative images than they were just twenty years ago; and over ten-thousand times the amount of negative images compared to seventy-five years ago.

The ears

Toxins get into your body through the ears, obviously, by anything you put in your ears as well as the sounds you hear. Sounds are vibrations and frequencies. Certain vibrations and frequencies sustain and cause life to grow. Certain vibrations and frequencies can cause degeneration and death. Certain music has been known to cause plants to grow at a faster rate, to be healthier and stronger. Other music has been shown to make plants wither and die. Think of all the sounds you are being exposed to that may have a negative effect on your physiology:

- The low hum of an air conditioner
- The computer running
- The alarm clock
- Certain kinds of "music"
- The washing machine, dryer, dish washer
- Your car engine
- Honking horns

If we stop for a moment and really listen to all the sounds that surround us, we find the majority are unnatural man-made frequencies. These frequencies go in through the ear and cause every cell in the body to be affected. If the frequency of the sound is not in tune with what nature intended, it can throw off the natural balance of the body. The simplest proof of this theory is how certain music, certain sounds and certain frequencies, cause a plant to either die or thrive. Think of the opera singer who hits a high note and shatters a crystal glass. That is how powerful vibrations, sounds, and frequencies are.

The electromagnetic field around the body

Medical science does not accept the notion that there is an electromagnetic field surrounding the body. However, we use electromagnetic energy, and science does admit that electromagnetic energy exists. Medical science claims there is no "scientific evidence" which proves that electromagnetic energy has any effect on the health or lack of health in the body. Remember that science has stated throughout history things that were not proven that have been later proven to be true. Science has proclaimed that there was "no scientific evidence" proving the earth was round; or that the earth revolved around the sun; or that nutrition had any effect on health; or that cigarettes were addictive. Science stated that anyone believing those things were heretics. The same is true now in relation to electromagnetic energy. Everything on this planet is made up of the same thing: atoms. All atoms resonate or vibrate at different frequencies. All atoms are made up of electrons, protons, and neutrons. Science admits that "energy" is what holds the electron in orbit around the nucleus. Science also admits that electrons, neutrons, and protons are made up of energy. Science admits that this energy can not be seen with the human eye or any accepted scientific equipment. Science also admits that it does not fully understand, and only theorizes about, these subatomic particles, or "energy." Yet, we see the effects of this "energy" all around us. Science can not see or explain how magnets work. However, you can easily see the effects of the magnetic field. Science can not explain how a satellite can beam electromagnetic energy that can pass through solid steel, be picked up by a radio transmitter, and magically turn into music. Think about it. If a satellite in the sky beams down electromagnetic energy twenty-four hours a day, seven days a week, and this energy is invisible, can not be detected, yet has the ability to pass through almost any material, and contains so much information that a "receiver" converts it into the music of an orchestra or images on a TV screen, isn't it possible that this energy is also hitting and passing through our bodies? Is it possible that this unnatural energy could have a negative impact on our bodies and our health? Something to think about. Awareness of electromagnetic energy is relatively new. It's really only been around in the last seventy-five years or so. Here are a few examples of the sources of unnatural electromagnetic energy that is bombarding our bodies every day:

- Satellites. There are dozens of satellites beaming down unnatural electromagnetic energy twenty-four hours a day, seven days a week.

- Radar. Radar stations for national defense and weather emit harmful electromagnetic energy twenty-four hours a day, seven days a week. It's interesting to note that many people believe that when these radar stations are put on maximum power during times of heightened security, a higher percentage of people feel ill, fatigued, and depressed. There is also the suggestion that those living close to these powerful radar towers have a higher chance of getting cancer, depression, and fatigue.

- Cell phone towers. These towers push out powerful energy waves on a consistent basis.

- Cell phones. When your cell phone is turned on it produces powerful unnatural electromagnetic energy, as well as drawing in all the cell phone tower energy. If the cell phone is within just a few feet of you, you are being affected.

- High tension power lines. These lines produce powerful amounts of negative energy affecting all living things in a large area around them.

- Electric wiring. Wiring encompasses our homes, our offices, our cars, any electronic device we carry, and is even buried under sidewalks and streets.

- Computers, televisions and radios. When these units are turned on, they emit large amounts of negative electromagnetic energy.

- Fluorescent lights. It is common knowledge that fluorescent lighting is an unnatural light source and can cause headaches, fatigue, and a weakening of the immune system. They also emit large doses of negative electromagnetic energy.

- Microwave ovens. The microwaves generated in these devices change the electromagnetic structure of whatever is in the oven into an unnatural, negative, life draining product. These devices also can leak the energy, adversely affecting those around it.

- Other people. Every person emits electromagnetic energy. A person's thoughts are also electromagnetic energy. The human body, especially the brain, is actually a very powerful transmitter and receiver of electromagnetic energy. This is why you feel good around some people and bad around others. Have you ever noticed that when certain people walk into a room, you can "sense" their presence? There are methods, which have not been accepted by the scientific community, which show the electromagnetic field around people and things. These technologies show the positive and negative effects of electromagnetic energy.

Another dynamic relating to electromagnetic energy is ions. There are positive and negative ions. Positively charged ions have an adverse effect on the body. Negatively charged ions have a positive, health-enhancing effect on the body. Running water such as a stream, waterfalls or the crashing waves of an ocean, emit large amounts of life-enhancing negative ions. The wind blowing through trees also emits these wonderful negative ions. This is why most people feel so much better when they are in these areas. Conversely, the wind blowing through tall buildings in cities, or an electric dryer, emits harmful positive ions. If you sit in a laundromat all day, it is very common for you to feel horrible and very fatigued. These harmful positive ions also can suppress your immune system. This electromagnetic chaos can not be avoided. However, it can be reduced, and there are simple things you can do to counteract the negative energy you are being exposed to.

The bottom line is that today we are putting more toxins in our body than ever before in history. And the trend is increasing. As this trend continues, people will continue to increase the number of times they get sick, the number of diseases they develop, and the severity and duration of these illnesses.

• • •

What comes out of the body

Our bodies, in normal function, produce toxins. This is fine, as long as our body's ability to eliminate these toxins is operating normally. Even if you put no toxins into your body, your body would still create waste material and toxins. All toxins created by the body or put into the body must be eliminated in order for us to be healthy. When toxins are allowed to accumulate they cause the immune system to be suppressed, and the body to become acidic. Accumulated toxins that have not been flushed out or eliminated allow the body to create an environment where illness and disease can flourish. We basically eliminate toxins through:

- The nose
- The mouth
- The urinary tract
- The colon
- The skin

The nose and mouth eliminate toxins primarily by use of the lungs. Our urinary tract eliminates toxins primarily through the kidneys and liver. The colon eliminates toxins primarily through the liver, the stomach and small intestine. The skin eliminates toxins primarily through perspiration. Most people today have excess accumulations of toxins and waste material in their bodies. The two main reasons for this are: 1) they are putting huge amounts of toxins in their body on a regular basis; 2) their elimination channels are clogged, slow, and sluggish.

When you put toxins in and your body creates toxins at a faster rate than you are eliminating those toxins, you have a build-up and accumulation of poisons and toxins in the body. For example, are your nasal and sinus cavities clear and mucus free? Do you breathe fully and deeply from your diaphragm, allowing your lungs to do their job fully? Do you regularly breathe aerobically and anaerobically? Do you sweat on a regular basis? Do you drink plenty of water, which allows all elimination channels to work more efficiently? Do you have three bowel movements per day? A few common things which slow the elimination process are:

- Antibiotics. If you have ever taken an antibiotic you have dramatically slowed your elimination potential via the colon. Antibiotics kill all the friendly bacteria in the intestine and colon. This allows unfriendly yeast, most notably candida, to grow abnormally and infest your digestive system. This candida yeast overgrowth slows digestion, increases gas, bloating and constipation, and itself creates an abnormal amount of toxins.

- Lotions and creams. Most people put lotions and creams all over their skin clogging the pores and suppressing the natural elimination process through the skin. This would include sunscreens, cosmetics, deodorants, and antiperspirants.

- Lack of body movement. Have you ever noticed when you take a dog for a walk, they poop? When you move your body as nature intended, you increase the elimination process. Since most people sit all day, their elimination cycles are suppressed. You should have three bowel movements per day. When you eat food, it goes through the digestion process and ends up in the colon ready for elimination.

The food in the colon begins to putrefy and become toxic. The longer it stays in the colon, the more toxic it becomes. If left long enough, these toxins begin to enter the bloodstream. This can turn into a serious medical condition resulting in death. Your body's elimination system must be working at optimal levels if you want to live without illness and disease.

Exercise

In simplistic terms, there are seven kinds of exercise:

1. *Slow rhythmic movement exercise.* This is mainly walking. The body is designed to walk, for long distances, and for long periods of time. The amount of walking in America varies per geographic area. New Yorkers tend to walk more than people living in Dallas. When you go to Europe or various other countries, people walk an average of eight to ten miles a day. In America people walk an average of close to one-tenth of a mile a day. And that is unbelievable. Walking is probably the most important form of exercise you can do, and the healthiest compared to driving, which increases stress. Now let's think about this for a moment. When you drive a car your stress levels go up dramatically, which means your body becomes acidic. When you go for a walk, not only are you getting the benefits of the exercise of the slow rhythmic movement, your lymph system is getting toxins out of your body, the body is moving and flowing beautifully, the energy is flowing through the meridians, and you are grounding your feet on the earth and getting the earth's magnetic energy to flow though your body, energizing your cells. You are also actually looking out and externalizing through your eyes at far away distances, which increases the electromagnetic energy in your body and makes the body more alkaline and less susceptible to disease. It also has a profound effect on your state of mind and happiness factor. The lack of walking causes the body's elimination channels to become slow and sluggish.

2. *Stretching.* Your body consists of muscles, tendons, and ligaments. If you lived in a natural setting, interacting with nature as we are designed, the natural activities you would be doing throughout your

day would cause the frequent stretching of your ligaments, muscles and tendons. Americans are the least flexible people in the world. Lack of flexibility allows for negative energy and toxins to accumulate in various parts of your body, allowing toxicity to build up.

3. *Resistance exercise.* This includes any form of movement where resistance is put against a muscle, and the muscle is required to push or pull against the resistance. The most common form of resistance training is weight lifting or the use of resistance machines. This is an unnatural form of exercise. Chimpanzees, as an example, are eight times stronger than a man, yet do not lift weights. Weight training can increase the size and strength of muscles, reshaping your body and making you look great. However, it generally only works with the muscles that are seen and does not address the majority of muscles that have no aesthetic value. It also does not address the strength of ligaments and tendons. This can create an imbalance, where some muscles are strong and abnormally large, and other muscles, ligaments and tendons are weak and disproportionate in size. Weight training does not increase flexibility—it actually reduces flexibility, thus hindering the flow of energy through the body. Nevertheless, doing any form of exercise is better than doing none at all.

4. *Postures.* There are certain exercise regimes where you are put into postures that are held for a period of time. The most commonly known is yoga. Keep in mind there are many forms of yoga. Not all kinds of yoga are posture based. Some yoga techniques are fluid and movement oriented. The benefits of postures are that they seem to help open up the natural energy channels in the body, and stimulate internal organs.

5. *Aerobic exercise.* Aerobic means "with air." Any form of exercise where you are breathing heavily but can still have a conversation is aerobic exercise. Aerobic exercise stimulates blood flow throughout the body, oxygenates the body and speeds the elimination of toxins.

6. *Anaerobic exercise.* Anaerobic means "without air." Any form of exercise where you are breathing so hard you can barely talk is anaerobic. The benefits are, generally, a tremendous stimulation of your entire

system because, in effect, you are putting the survival of every cell in your body at risk because of the lack of oxygen. This is very helpful in "reprogramming the body" and allowing the body to increase its elimination of toxins and stop any cellular activity that was abnormal.

7. *Cellular exercise.* At this time there is only one form of exercise that actually affects, in a positive way, every cell in the body simultaneously. Jumping on a trampoline has been shown to stimulate and strengthen every cell in the body. This unique form of exercise dramatically increases the movement through the lymph system, stimulates every cell's elimination of toxins, and increases the strength and vitality of every cell in the body.
   The major benefits of cellular exercise include:

- *Increase oxygen to the cells.* Oxygen is needed for life. Most people are deficient in the amount of oxygen they have throughout their bodies. Viruses and cancer, for example, can not exist in an oxygen rich environment. An oxygen rich body is an alkaline body. An alkaline body is a body where disease and illness can not exist.

- *Movement of lymph fluid.* The lymphatic system is an important element in the elimination process. Most Americans have a lymphatic system that is dangerously clogged and sluggish. Moving the body as it was intended increases the movement of lymph fluid through the body, assisting with the elimination of toxins.

- *Cell stimulation.* Every cell in the body produces toxic waste. Every cell in the body needs stimulation in order for the toxic waste to be eliminated. Every cell in the body needs stimulation to remain healthy and thrive in a normal way. If a cell does not eliminate the toxic waste it produces and does not receive stimulation, it can begin to act in an abnormal way. Cells could degenerate and die or begin to grow abnormally in an out of control manner, causing tumors, cancer, or the degeneration of vital organs in the body.

- *Opening of energy channels.* Energy flows through our body. Just like blood flows through the veins, electromagnetic energy flows through channels in our body. When these channels are blocked or congested, energy does not flow efficiently. This energy gives life and vitality to the cells; without it the cells do not receive what is needed, causing abnormalities, suppression of the immune system, and turning the body acidic, making it susceptible to illness. Exercise helps to keep these channels open.

- *Releasing of tension and stress.* Stress is the silent killer. Stress can be defined many ways. In simplistic terms, stress is holding on to negative energy. When negative energy is being held, it can lodge itself into various parts of the body. This can cause muscles to be tight and the body to become acidic. Exercise breaks up this stress and tension, and can allow it to leave the body.

I have already told you how stress is ultimately the cause of all disease. When something stresses us, our body turns from a natural state of alkaline pH to acidic. When it's acidic, disease can grow. Stress suppresses our immune system and makes us weaker and more susceptible to infections, germs, bacteria and viruses. When our immune system is weak, we can not naturally defend against these invaders and we get sick. So the question is, what are the stressors and how can we eliminate them?

Rest

Without proper rest, the cells are not given the opportunity to recharge and rejuvenate. Tired cells can not eliminate toxins efficiently. It is also during rest that most healing takes place. Most people do not get enough rest, and the rest they do get is not full and deep. There are three elements of proper rest:

1. *The time in which you rest.* The most optimum time for the body to rest is when the sun is no longer shining. Ideally, a person would rest and sleep when the sun goes down and arise when the sun comes up. This is the natural cycle. However, most people's lifestyles do not allow this. Therefore they are resting and sleeping at non-optimal times. Each week a lunar cycle occurs starting at sundown every Friday ending at sundown every Saturday. This time period is absolutely the most ideal time for the body to recharge and rejuvenate.

2. *The amount of hours you rest.* Although every person is different, it appears that every person operates better when getting eight hours of

sleep. People operate worse if they receive fewer hours or more hours. The majority of people sleep less than eight hours, and then try to catch up by occasionally sleeping more hours. This practice does not allow optimal recharging and rejuvenation of the cells in your body.

3. *Rest and sleep should be deep.* Most people toss and turn at night. The ideal situation is that you virtually do not move for the entire sleep time. When sleep is full and deep, brainwave activity can occur, which stimulates the healing process throughout the body. A person who snores wakes themselves up an average of 300 times per night. A person who snores never gets into the deepest levels of sleep, and thus their body is never operating at optimal efficiency.

There is a difference between sleep and rest. The body can rest without going to sleep. Most people never take a "rest" during the day. The common pattern of waking up, working all day non-stop, going to bed late, never getting a full deep eight hours of peaceful sleep, results in a body that slowly begins to break down and never has a chance to heal and recharge. If you were to take a battery powered device and leave it on until the battery died, and compare that to turning the device on for a period of time then off for a period of time, repeating this process several times, you would find the battery life can be as high as twice as long as non-stop usage. The body is very much like a battery. The body operates almost identically, utilizing electric current throughout. It must be given a chance to rest. If a person did nothing else but get proper rest and sleep, their energy levels would skyrocket and the amount of illness and disease they experience would go down dramatically.

Your thoughts

Thoughts are things. Your body is in fact a very powerful electromagnetic transmitter and receiver of energy. Every thought you have can have a powerful impact on the cells in your body. Positive high vibration thoughts can rid your body of disease. Negative stressful low vibration thoughts can give your body disease. Science does not believe that thoughts can have any profound effect on your health. Medical science believes that thoughts could never alone cure or cause disease. However, it is interesting to point out that medical science can not dispute the "placebo" effect. The placebo effect is when a person is given a "placebo," which is in effect nothing, yet their disease is cured. This occurs because the patient believes that what he is taking will cure the disease. His thoughts basically cause the cure. This happens in as many as 40 percent of the cases. Imagine, up to 40 percent of the time a person with a dreaded disease cures himself with his own thoughts! Yet, remember our friends at the FDA who say that only a drug can cure a disease.

Thoughts can heal, but they can also cause sickness and disease. Stress, which could be defined as negative thoughts, cause the body to become acidic, thus creating the environment for illness and disease. These negative thoughts can be conscious or unconscious in nature. Many of these negative thoughts are trapped in stressful or traumatic incidences from our past. Several prominent doctors have found that the vast majority of people with cancer have an incident in their past that caused tremendous grief. Individuals who have heart attacks are found to have suppressed anger. It is interesting to note the correlation between certain emotions and certain diseases. The stress of living in today's environment is higher than at any time in history. Driving a car, for example, raises stress levels in the body up to 1,000 times normal levels. When a person is driving a car combined with talking on a cell phone, stress levels can go as high as 5,000 times the norm. Walking, conversely, actually reduces stress. Worrying about money, arguing with relatives, friends and co-workers, watching scary gruesome movies and television shows, reading the news, all increase stress levels dramatically. The good news is this can be reversed. Doctor Coldwell of Germany has the highest cancer success rate in the country, treating over 35,000 mostly terminal cancer patients. Without drugs or surgery, but rather by using techniques to reduce stress, in effect correcting a person's thoughts, he has cured more people of cancer than any person in German history. Dr. Norman Cousins' *The Anatomy of an Illness* documents how, by laughing and reducing stress, without drugs or surgery, cancer was put in complete remission. Earl Nightingale discovered what he called "The strangest secret: You become what you think about." Positive thoughts and low amounts of stress create an alkaline pH in the body, meaning you virtually can not get sick.

Negative thoughts and emotions and high levels of stress cause the body to become acidic, leading to illness and disease.

What you say

Words have power. Most people speak words that increase body stress and turn the body's pH from alkaline to acidic. Words can change the way we think and feel. Researchers have concluded that speaking the correct form of words and thinking the correct thoughts actually changes a person's DNA.

Of all of these things, I believe that the most important are what we think and what we say. If you look at people today around the world who have no disease and no illness, there are virtually no common denominators. Nobody can look to a person's genetic disposition. You can't look to a person's diet because they vary so greatly. Some of these people smoke, some of them eat monkeys raw, some of them eat dairy products, some of them are vegetarians, some of them do exercise, others simply walk. They generally all do sleep very well, but the most obvious common denominator is how they think and how they talk. They are very positive, optimistic individuals, they don't take life very seriously, and they don't care about that much. They are optimistic and they are light-hearted. They greet each day in a spirit of thankfulness. Attitude really makes the difference, thoughts do affect the body, and thoughts can dramatically affect your health.

From a biological standpoint, what does this really mean? Think of it this way. The body has what is known as the immune system. The immune system fights off any imbalance or disease, virus, germs and bacteria. If your body's immune system is strong and you happen to catch any bacteria or virus, your body fights it off and you never even notice that you were exposed or had that particular virus or bacteria or germ. When your immune system is very weak, you are susceptible to showing the symptoms of succumbing to that particular virus or bacteria.

So the summary, in very general, very simplistic terms is this:

The reason why you are sick is because you are putting more toxins and chemicals in your body. Those toxins and chemicals are not coming out of your body because you are not eliminating things like you should. We are exercising more but we are not walking, and walking is the major form of exercise that gives you the most health benefits. We are not resting enough, so our body doesn't have a chance to rejuvenate and recharge. Our thoughts are more negative because of the images we are getting from television, magazines, newspapers and movies. Think about the kids' games that they are playing and how horrific those images are. The sounds we are hearing are not life enhancing, but are actually having a powerful adverse affect on our physiology—turning our body from alkaline to acid. And we are being bombarded by more electronic chaos from cell phones, microwaves, satellite waves, electronic devices, computers, televisions, etc. We drive more than ever before and, due to that, our stress levels keep going up and up, causing our bodies to become more acidic and giving us a whole environment which is conducive to sickness and disease. Our immune systems are being suppressed and we are becoming more susceptible to illness. Specifically, the drugs that we are taking are making our immune systems weaker, and are putting so many toxins in our bodies that they are in fact causing many additional illnesses.

You'll notice that every major illness that we face today, those that most people are popping drugs for, are not in fact caused by bacteria or viruses. We aren't catching them. We develop them in our body. They are actually self-inflicted illnesses. If your body's immune system is strong and healthy, when you are exposed to the viruses and bacteria which we all are every single day, your body would simply handle them and you wouldn't even notice them. If you did have a scratchy throat, if you did have some sniffles or a cough, it would maybe last a few hours or a day at most. You wouldn't have to take any drug, your body would handle it and deal with it and become stronger because of it. That's the natural way your body reacts. We forget that many of the symptoms we have are actually our body's own defense mechanisms working properly, so we go out and take drugs and try to suppress them.

A good example is a fever. If you have a fever, the body is raising its temperature to fight off some danger. But what we do is, we go out and take something to reduce our fever, allowing the invaders to take over.

The problem with medical procedures, and the problem with drugs and surgery is that they all try to solve or eliminate a symptom. They never ask, "What's the cause?" If you have a fever, don't say you need to get rid of the fever. Ask yourself what's causing the fever. Keep asking and keep asking and keep asking that question. By eliminating the symptoms, you just suppress the real cause of the problem, thus causing it to get worse. If you are driving your car and your oil light goes on, you wouldn't say "my oil light's on; I need to get my oil light to go off. Oh, I know what I'll do, I'll unscrew the bulb. Ah, now the oil light is no longer illuminated." You haven't solved the problem, have you? You got rid of a symptom. There is no more illumination of the oil light. But the reason that light went on is still there. You may drive that car for another few weeks before it seizes up on you. Your body is the same way. If you have a headache, you shouldn't say, "Let me eliminate the pain of the headache." You should ask yourself what's causing your body to do that, and find the cause. When you do this, you are addressing the root cause of problems and not just treating symptoms.

Medical science, medical doctors, drugs and surgery only treat symptoms. The question that always comes up for me is: Is there a place for drugs and surgery? And the answer is: Absolutely yes! I have to applaud the medical community because they have developed the best methods to date of keeping a person alive in the event of a trauma, accident or emergency situation. If we go with the theory that we always ask, "what's the cause," and not just treat the symptom, then we can use drugs and surgery as they should be used. Here's an example:

I'm walking in my garden and I step on a nail. I rush to the emergency room and say, "Quick, I stepped on a nail. It was a rusty nail. I'm bleeding, and I'm in pain. Help!" The doctor says that you may have some infection and gives you some ointment that will kill the bacteria to make sure you don't get an infection. He gives you some type of drug that will stop the bleeding and sews you up with a surgical procedure to handle the wound. The reason that is acceptable is because the cause of my problem was stepping on a nail. We have addressed the cause. It's not going to repeat itself. We know what the cause is. Now let's handle the symptoms.

If I was in a car crash and my kidney was ripped open by the metal of the crushed vehicle, rush me to the emergency room and handle my symptoms. Don't ask: "Hmm, I wonder what caused this? Let's go for the cause." I can tell you what the cause is. The cause is a piece of metal ripped my skin open and punctured my kidney; please use drugs and surgery and save my life. Handle the symptoms. The symptoms are, "I am bleeding profusely, I'm about to die." Handling the symptoms is good in that situation.

But if a person has cancer you don't say: "Hmm, cancer cells...let me cut them out, let me shoot them full of radiation, let me give them some drugs that may kill them." Ask yourself why cancer is growing in the body. The answer is: The body is acidic. What's causing the body to be acidic? Let's find out what is going into the body, what is going out of the body, what the person thinks, how he is exercising, how he is resting and what he is saying, and let's turn this around in a very simple way and then the cancer goes away. We reduce stress, we strengthen the immune system, the body becomes alkaline, and disease can't exist.

The conclusion, then, is that people get sick because:

- We are putting too many toxins in our body and not flushing the toxins out fast enough. Meaning our body is toxic.

- We are not putting enough of the necessary nutrients into our body, and the nutrients that are going in are not being absorbed. This means we are nutritionally deficient.

Since all matter consists ultimately of energy, in simplistic terms the cause of all disease is energetic imbalance. This can also be defined as "stress." When this occurs, we are susceptible to germs, bacteria, and viruses, and our body prematurely ages and develops a vast array of diseases and medical problems.

C H A P T E R   6

How to Never Get Sick Again

You can call this chapter: "How to Cure Every Disease"; "How to Live Healthy and Disease Free Forever"; "How to be Young Forever"; "How to Have Dynamic, Vibrant Health." You can call this chapter anything you want, but basically this chapter will give you the information to potentially eliminate any illness or disease you may currently have, and prevent any illness and disease in the future. This information will also allow you to potentially slow down and even reverse the aging process. Keep in mind that I am not a medical doctor. If you are currently being treated by a medical doctor make sure they are informed as to what you are doing. I can not diagnose or treat anyone's medical conditions. I present this for educational purposes only. This information is strictly my opinion and based on the information currently available. I believe everything to be true and accurate.

Right now, you either have some known illness or disease such as cancer, diabetes, etc., or you claim to be "healthy." If you claim to be healthy, you probably still experience the normal occasional headaches, aches and pains, fatigue, indigestion, colds and flus, heartburn, etc. So-called healthy people believe that these occasional medical conditions are "normal." They are not. A healthy person has little, if any, body odor, they have no bad breath, no foot odor, their urine and stool do not smell, they sleep soundly, they have no skin rashes or dandruff, they are not depressed or stressed, they rarely if ever get colds, flus, heartburn, aches and pains. Truly healthy people are full of energy and vitality, and never have to take any nonprescription or prescription drug because they never have any symptoms that would require them to take a drug. So, in reality every one of you reading this book is unhealthy to some degree. I can assure you that if you continue to do what you always have, your physical health will slowly begin to deteriorate, you will get more sickness and diseases, and your energy levels will continually go down.

Some people always ask me if all I say is true; how did "Aunt Millie" live to be eighty-five? First, I say that I would like to offer my condolences for Aunt Millie's premature death. It is sad to see someone die so young. You see, I believe that the human body, like all mammals, should live to be well over 100 years old. When you compare the life spans of virtually all mammals, they live well in excess of what would be the equivalent of 120 human years. So, dying at eighty-five to me is dying young. Secondly, Aunt Millie lived the first half of her life where the amount of toxins being put into the body was a fraction of what it is today. I hear a lot about the alleged fact that we are living longer than ever before. This is categorically not true. Yes, it is true that people lie in nursing homes and hospital beds hooked up to life support devices that keep the physical body alive for years, but realistically these people are not living. The statistics on life span are fraudulent and false. The fact of the matter is a person 100 years old should be strong, flexible, full of life and energy, and have the physical capacity of what the average forty-year-old person has. It is amusing to me when you hear the American Medical Association classify someone in their fifties as being "older," and someone in their sixties as being "old." The most amazing part of this is that it is assumed that as you get older, it is "normal" to be on some type of medication. This simply is not true.

The bottom line is that you are either: a) very sick; b) somewhat sick; or c) about to get sick.

It is hard to find a truly healthy person. The good news is there is a way out. Let's examine where you are right now. You are full of toxins. You are also deficient in necessary nutrients. The energy in your body is not flowing properly. Many of your systems are not operating at optimal levels. You either notice severe symptoms, or you have mild symptoms that you classify as normal. What can we do to: a) eradicate any and all symptoms you have, thus "curing" the disease or illness, and b) prevent any illness or disease from starting, thus giving you a tremendous increase in energy, vitality, and vibrant dynamic health? The first thing I would recommend is that you seek proper healthcare from a professional healthcare provider who does not use drugs or surgery. Since every person is different, and every condition is different, you need to have a knowledgeable person examine you and give you appropriate care. Keep in mind that all healthcare providers have different backgrounds and experiences, and may have different opinions about the course of action that is best for you. It is wise to get several opinions from several people.

The big question I get often is: How do I find a good alternative, all-natural healthcare provider? This is an excellent question. Unfortunately, these healthcare practitioners can not advertise because the FDA is looking for people who are curing disease without drugs and surgery, and if the FDA becomes aware of these people, history shows that the FDA or FTC will drive these healthcare practitioners out of business. A simple way to find someone good in your area is to go down to your local health food store and ask who they recommend. On my website, www.naturalcures.com, I have a private member area where you can be provided with recommendations of people in your area that have excellent track records in using all-natural therapies. Generally speaking, healthcare providers who practice homeopathy, acupuncture, chiropractic medicine, herbology and nutritional therapy are all good places to start. I myself have been treated by over 200 natural healthcare providers from around the world. Is one better than the other? Yes. They are also, in many cases, very different in their approach. Do they all provide some benefit? I believe so. Do some treatments and therapies work faster and more completely than others? Yes. However, the one that works best for me may not work best for you. Everyone is different, every situation and condition is different, and the same treatment may have varying results with each person. You have to take responsibility for your own health. No one knows it all. No one, including the pharmaceutical industry and medical doctors, has a monopoly on the truth. So the first step is to seek out alternative, all-natural healthcare providers, and start experiencing for yourself the benefits you'll enjoy without drugs and surgery.

If you choose not to seek appropriate individualized care, or even if you do, I believe that doing the following things can potentially cure disease and illness that you may currently have (provided, of course, that the condition is not past the point of no return), and prevent illness and disease from ever occurring. These recommendations are also the best way to slow, or potentially reverse, the aging process, making you look and feel younger than you have in years.

In general terms the way to eradicate any and all illness and disease that you may have, prevent illness and disease from occurring in the future, and slowdown or potentially reverse the aging process is to do the following:

- Eliminate the toxins that have built up in your system. You are loaded with toxins. The only question is, how much. You absolutely must get these toxins out of your body if you want to cure and prevent illness and disease. Getting the toxins out of your body can immediately increase energy, help you lose weight, eliminate depression and anxiety, and potentially reverse most illnesses and disease. The basic cleanses that you should do are: a) a colon cleanse; b) a liver cleanse; c) a gallbladder cleanse; d) a lung cleanse; e) a fat tissue cleanse; and f) a lymphatic cleanse. At my website, www.naturalcures.com, I give you my specific recommendations of how and where to do these cleanses.

- Clean up and repair the damaged energy field around and in your body.

- Open up the energy channels in your body.

- Stop, or at least reduce, the amount of toxins coming into your body. In today's world it is impossible to totally eliminate putting toxins in your body, but we can dramatically reduce the amount of toxins that go into our system.

- Stop, reduce or neutralize the negative electromagnetic energy attacking your energy field and body.

- Put in your body an abundance of life-giving nutrients that you are deficient in.

- Put in your body food that is full of lifeforce energy.

- Eliminate trapped thought patterns that are charged with negative energy.
- Use your thoughts to alkalize the body instead of acidifying the body.

The following is a list of my specific recommendations that achieve the above results. As I mentioned in an earlier chapter, the FDA and FTC and other organizations use censorship on a regular basis so that people do not have access to this information. Even though my First Amendment rights allow me "free speech," the FTC has ordered me not to tell you of any specific products that I recommend. Yes, censorship is alive and well in America. Yes, my First Amendment rights have been taken away. Yes, if I say what I want to say and exercise my constitutional First Amendment right to free speech, the FTC could prosecute me, imprison me, and confiscate and burn all of my books! I know it sounds like Nazi Germany, but this is true and happening now to people all over this country. Suppression by the government of the free flow of information is at an all time high and getting worse. So, I can not give you the specific names of products I recommend, nor can I give you in this book the names of the companies that sell these products. However, if you go to my website and go to the private member area, you can e-mail me and I will be happy to give you my personal recommendations. Keep in mind, I do not sell any of the products I recommend. I am not paid by the companies to recommend their products. I am not compensated in any way if you choose to buy the products that I recommend. I only sell books and information. And I donate much of the profits that I earn to organizations that promote health and freedom. If this is as outrageous to you as it is to me, please go to my website www.naturalcures.com and become a member. Being a member will allow us to flood the politicians with mail so that our freedom of health choices can be brought back.

Do not be overwhelmed with this list. I recommend you look over the list and try to do as much as you can to the degree you feel comfortable. Add one or two recommendations weekly. Remember, doing even a little can make a huge difference in how you feel physically. The list is not necessarily in order from most important to least important. A recommendation close to the end of the list could be the most important and have the most profound effect on you. However, generally speaking, based on my experience and observations, the recommendations at the top have more significant results for most people than those closer to the end. Each of these recommendations can easily take an entire book to explain in detail. As a matter of fact, on each one of these recommendations there are actually many books written on just that one particular subject. I have read most of the books or have interviewed the authors themselves as I conducted my research. This is why I am making the recommendations. Many of you may be interested in learning more about an individual subject. On my website I give you a list of the best books that, in most cases, cover just one single subject. This book, as you are aware by now, covers dozens of subjects. I encourage you to call us and order the books that you are interested in as you continue to learn the secret truths of health and vitality. With that said, all of these things are very important and can have dramatic affects on your health.

1. **See natural healthcare providers on a regular basis**

   When you have a car that you love and cherish, you keep it clean on the inside and out. You do not wait for the car to make funny noises or stop running; you instead bring the car in on a regular basis for maintenance. This regular maintenance is designed to prevent any problems from occurring. Your body should be treated in a similar fashion. You should be seeing various natural healthcare providers from a variety of disciplines, even when you don't experience symptoms. Seeing more than one person is valuable so that all bases are covered.

2. **Stop taking nonprescription and prescription drugs**

   If you are taking drugs of any kind, do not do this step without consulting your physician. Remember, drugs are poisons. This includes vaccines. Although opinions vary, many experts believe that vaccines are the number one cause of deaths and disease in children. Vaccines are some of the most toxic things you can put in your body.

   Last year over 250,000 Americans died by taking the proper dosage of prescription and nonprescription drugs. It is estimated that millions had to receive medical treatment because of the horrible side effects from taking prescription and nonprescription drugs. It is also estimated that tens of millions will develop long-term medical conditions because they took nonprescription and prescription drugs. In my opinion, drugs should only be taken in the most severe cases.

3. Energetic rebalancing

Frequency generators have been around for decades. Royal Rife was using frequencies in the 1920s and 1930s to cure cancer. Today there are several machines using frequencies to balance out a person's energy, thus eliminating the energetic frequency of the imbalance or disease. When the frequency of the disease you have has been neutralized, the disease goes away. These machines absolutely, 100 percent allow the body to virtually cure all diseases. They are fast, painless and inexpensive. They are also outlawed by the FDA. Individual practitioners using these machines never publicly claim that they cure anything for fear that the FDA will prosecute these people for using an unlicensed medical device and curing people without the legally approved drugs. These machines include the Intero, Vegatest, Dermatron, and others. The most advanced technology that I know of is used by a man in Southern California who treats many well known celebrities. His technology is so advanced that, no matter where you are in the world, he can have his computerized frequency machine monitoring you twenty-four hours a day, seven days per week, constantly balancing the energetic frequencies in your body. I personally have been using this technology for the last seven years, and I have never in that time been sick. When everyone around me had a serious cold, I got the sniffles for about two hours. When all my friends got the flu, I never experienced a single symptom. I highly recommend you read the book *Sanctuary* to get the full story on this revolutionary technology. Here's what some others have to say about this program.

Dr. Wayne W. Dyer, bestselling author of *Wisdom of the Ages*; lecturer; spiritual teacher:

"In regard to Stephen Lewis, EMC², and the AIM Program: Everything is energy. Everything and everyone has a frequency.

Those frequencies that are out of balance with our natural harmony can be identified and removed. I know this to be true. I have seen the Sanctuary process at work. I practice it daily. My entire family participates in the AIM Program, and I have seen wonderful results. This is real, it is transforming, it is true healing, and it is a giant step into the inevitable future where each of us is our own personal, transcendental, and totally enlightened healer. I have found that in my higher self, and so can you. It is available now."

Linda Gray, actress, Goodwill Ambassador on Women's Issues to the United Nations:

"I have used this technology for years. It is the most glorious gift that anyone could receive."

Courtney Cox Arquette, actress:

"I've been fortunate enough to have participated in Energetic Balancing® for over three years. I don't know what I would do without it. I don't believe anyone can afford not to be a part of it."

To order the book *Sanctuary*, call 800-931-4721, or go to www.naturalcures.com.

4. **Check your body pH**

   Dr. Morter discovered a specific technique for testing the pH of your saliva and urine. You can do this test with a simple piece of pH paper. It takes less than five minutes. Do this test once a week or as often as you like. If your body pH is too acidic, you know you need to do some things to correct the out of balance state. If your body pH is in the proper alkaline state, you know that the chance of you getting cancer or other diseases is almost zero. This is a great way for you to see first hand how these various techniques are benefiting you. The complete instructions for this test are on my website www.naturalcures.com.

5. **Eat more fresh organic fruits and vegetables**

   You don't have to be a vegetarian to be healthy. I have never seen any real, convincing evidence that vegetarians are healthier or live longer than people who eat animal products. However, the healthiest people absolutely eat a large amount of fresh, organic, raw, uncooked fruits and vegetables. If you were to do just one thing, I would tell you to eat four pieces of fresh fruit per day and two big raw salads full of vegetables. If you changed nothing else in your diet, but just added those two things, many medical conditions would disappear. Ideally, the fruits and vegetables should be organic and uncooked, but cooked non-organic fruits and vegetables are better than none at all.

6. **Do a candida elimination program**

   If you have ever taken a single dose of antibiotics any time in your life, you have a candida yeast overgrowth in your body. This overgrowth is most common in the intestine, but can infiltrate your entire body. This overgrowth can be a cause of virtually every symptom you can imagine—headaches, gas bloating, indigestion, heartburn, nausea, allergies asthma, fibromyalgia, arthritis, diabetes, constipation, yeast infections, dandruff, acne, bad breath, fatigue, depression, stress, and on and on. Doing a program that eliminates the excess candida from your body is one of the backbones of good health. The most common side effect of excess candida is the inability to lose weight. People who eliminate excess candida virtually always lose massive amounts of weight without trying. Candida also causes food cravings and can make you eat when you're not hungry. When candida is normalized, a person's appetite can be dramatically reduced so that you're just simply not that hungry.

7. **Buy a juice machine and use it**

   Animals don't own juice machines, but animals have not loaded their bodies with the amount of toxins we have. They use their bodies as they were designed, unlike us, and they eat raw, uncooked food full of living enzymes and packed with nutrition and life force energy. Our food supply today is dramatically depleted of vital vitamins and minerals. Organic produce has up to ten times the vitamin and minerals as non-organic, and has none of the poison residues of the chemical fertilizers, pesticides and fungicides. Even so, because the soil is so depleted, organic produce still has less nutritional value than the same produce had fifty years ago. You would have to eat ten times the amount of produce today to even come close to the nutritional value of food fifty years ago. Therefore, it is absolutely impossible to get the amount of vitamins, minerals, and enzymes that you need by simply eating food. And remember, because of all of the drugs and toxins you have ingested, your ability to absorb these nutrients is dramatically reduced. Even if you ate only raw, uncooked organic fruits, vegetables, nuts and seeds, your body would have major nutritional deficiencies. The absolute best way to correct this problem is to buy a good juice machine and make fresh juice using organic fruits and vegetables. Drinking three to four glasses of fresh juice gives your body a huge amount of living enzymes, as well as vitamins and minerals in the natural state and in the proportion that nature intended.

8. **Do alphabiotics**

   Alphabiotics is a very powerful treatment that dramatically reduces stress in the body, makes one think clearer, and dramatically reduces muscle tension and pain. It is excellent for increasing energy flow throughout the body and keeping the body's posture correct. For more information go to www.naturalcures.com.

9. **Get natural sunlight**

   Go for a walk in the sun! Your body needs sunlight. Do not use sunglasses or sun screens. The sun enters through the eyes and stimulates energy in the entire body. Thirty minutes a day, minimum, in the sun promotes incredible health benefits. Remember, it is the sun that creates growth in plants. The solar energy from sun can be very alkalizing to the body; it reduces depression, and strengthens your immune system. Don't be misled by the medical establishment. The sun is good for you and its absolutely needed.

10. **Do a colon cleanse**

    For my personal recommendations of the best cleanses, go to www.naturalcures.com.

11. **Do a liver and gallbladder cleanse**

    For my personal recommendations of the best cleanses, go to www.naturalcures.com.

12. **Don't drink tap water**

All tap water is poisonous. All tap water is loaded with chlorine and chlorine by-products. Chlorine scars your arteries and, along with hydrogenated oil and homogenized dairy products, causes heart disease. Most tap water also has fluoride, which is one of the most poisonous and disease causing agents you can put in your body. Do not drink or use tap water for any reason except for washing your floor.

You need to drink water, and the water must be pure Water is instrumental not only in flushing and nourishing the body, but also in keeping it hydrated and pH balanced. I recommend drinking a minimum of six large glasses of water per day. I recommend a specific water purifier and specific bottled waters. Not all water filters or purifiers do an equally effective job. Some are much better than others. Not all bottled waters are equally pure and hydrating. Some are much better than others. Go to www.naturalcures.com for my personal recommendations.

13. **Eat an apple a day**

14. **Take coral calcium**

The Federal Trade Commission forbids me to say anything about coral calcium. For the truth, go to www.naturalcures.com.

15. **Take a whole food supplement**

Your body is deficient in vitamins, minerals, enzymes, and cofactors. That is a fact. There is no way that you can get all the nutrients you need by eating food. You would have to eat ten to twenty times the amount of food as you are now, and it would all have to be organic. There simply is no way you are getting the nutrients you need. Having the proper amount of vitamins, minerals, enzymes and cofactors allows your body to operate as it was designed. The best way to get this needed nutrition is by making fresh juice at home. But I also suggest buying a whole food concentrate nutritional supplement. Your product should not contain any chemical of synthetic nutrients, but only organic, raw concentrated food sources. For my personal recommendations, go to www.naturalcures.com.

16. **Buy a shower filter**

    You absorb more toxins by taking one shower than by drinking six glasses of water. Your skin absorbs the water from your shower or bath. A hot shower produces steam and that turns many of the chemicals in the water into poisonous gases. These gases are inhaled or absorbed through the skin. A good shower filter removes most of the toxins in the water. Use one and you'll never have a bad hair day again. For my personal recommendations go to www.naturalcures.com.

17. **Use magnetic finger and toe rings**

    These are inexpensive and easy to use. Simply wear this specially designed magnetic ring on the small finger of each hand, and if you want even more benefit, wear the toe brace on each foot. These are worn when you sleep. The health benefits seem to be almost unbelievable. This device appears to radically slow the aging process and, in most cases, appears to reverse the aging process; people report looking and feeling younger as time goes on. These are absolutely amazing. For information on where these are available go to www.naturalcures.com.

18. **Use a rebounder**

    A rebounder is a mini trampoline. Simply using this device for five minutes a day can provide more cellular benefit than almost any other form of exercise. A rebounder stimulates every cell in the body simultaneously. It stimulates the immune system and is incredibly effective at cleansing toxins out of the cells. It promotes and stimulates all major organs and glands, strengthens the immune system and dramatically strengthens and tones the muscles, tendons, and ligaments. A truly spectacular and incredibly quick form of exercise.

19. **Get treated by an bioenergetic synchronization technique practitioner**

    Dr. Morter invented this technique. He has trained thousands of people in this treatment. This technique is painless and takes only a few minutes. It is an incredibly effective way of rebalancing the body, reducing or eliminating pain or trauma, and is very powerful in helping your body go from acid to alkaline. For more information go to www.naturalcures.com.

20. **Only eat organic, kosher meat and poultry**

This subject is incredibly complex. Oprah Winfrey had a show devoted to the meat industry, and was sued for expressing her opinions. She won. Any meat or poultry that is not organic and kosher is incredibly toxic. Generally speaking, here are the differences:

- A conventional animal has been genetically modified in breeding, thus becoming an animal that could never occur naturally.

- An organic animal has genetics that have not been modified by man and is in its most natural state.

- A conventional animal is injected with growth hormone and antibiotics, meaning that the meat we consume is then loaded with these drugs.

- An organic animal is given no drugs, so its meat is drug free.

- A conventional animal is not allowed to roam freely or exercise normally, thus creating an incredibly toxic animal that is unnaturally obese and diseased.

- An organic animal is allowed to roam naturally, grows at its normal rate, and is not loaded with toxins or diseased.

- A conventional animal is fed an unnatural diet of chemicals and feed that it would never eat naturally. Conventional cows, for example, are also fed ground up cow parts, pig parts, goat parts, and horse parts. Many of these

- A grass-fed organic cow eats grass as it would in nature, and the grass has not been laced with chemical fertilizers, herbicides, and pesticides.

ground up animal parts are from diseased, sick animals that are not fit for human consumption. Keep in mind the cow is a vegetarian and is not designed to be eating ground up diseased animals.

- A conventional animal is slaughtered by being shot in the head with a bolt. The animal experiences incredible pain and trauma. Adrenaline, which is highly poisonous, permeates the animal's tissue. The blood, which is loaded with toxins, also permeates the issue. The trauma causes the energy field in and around the animal to become highly negative. The animal usually dies in its own urine and feces.

- An organic animal, that is also kosher, is killed in the most humane way possible, by slicing its throat. The animal experiences no pain, is immediately drained of all blood, its internal organs are inspected to make sure the animal is 100 percent healthy, and the tissue is salted to draw out any blood and kill any bacteria.

- A conventional animal is usually aged, which means the animal flesh is hung in a dark room and allowed to rot. A green mold covers the rotting animal flesh. This green toxic mold is bacteria that tenderizes the meat, but also fills the meat with more toxic poisons.

- Organic kosher meat is not aged.

Many conventional meat and poultry products are sprayed with dangerous chemicals to kill bacteria. Some are irradiated, wiping out the natural life force energy and, as evidenced by Kirlian photography, leaving the energy field around the meat highly toxic to humans.

When I learned about this, I decided to eat only kosher organic meat. For thirty days, every day, I ate some kosher organic meat. I tried to monitor if I felt any difference. I could not detect anything specific or dramatic. I wasn't convinced that it was such a big deal. I decided to throw a barbeque and invited several of my friends over to my home. I went to the butcher and bought the absolute best, highest quality steaks made—conventional, Black Angus aged steaks. The best money can buy. I cooked the steaks and served them to my guests. Each person raved about how delicious and tender the steaks were. Some said they were the best they had ever eaten. I took one bite of mine and felt very odd. It was as if I was eating some "bad meat." I looked around at everyone else devouring their steaks and enjoying the delicious flavor. I asked my friend to taste my steak. He loved it. So I took another bite. As I chewed and swallowed the meat I began to feel funny. Perspiration started on my forehead, I got pale, and my stomach felt very nauseous. I excused myself, went to the bathroom and threw up.

What had occurred was that for thirty days I only ate pure nontoxic, undiseased meat. Eating this highly toxic meat caused me to get sick, because I had eaten only clean meat for so long my body had immediately rejected the toxins. This is why people in Mexico, for example, can drink the diseased toxic water and show no signs of illness. But if an American were to drink the same water, they would get violently ill. Your body does create a tolerance to poisons.

The bottom line is, chicken, duck, lamb, beef, and goat are all fine as long as it is organic and kosher. It is hard to find organic kosher products in stores. On my website www.naturalcures.com you can find out where this is available.

21. **Get a magnetic mattress pad**

The earth, at one time, had a magnetic level (called gauss) of 4.0. Today the earth's gauss is .04. Sleeping on a mattress pad filled with magnets stimulates energy flowing through the body as nature intended. It has been said to alleviate pain, slow the aging process, increase energy, and helps alkalize the body. There are many good pads on the market. For my personal recommendations, go to www.naturalcures.com.

22. **Do not drink canned or bottled juice**

23. **Get 15 colonics in 30 days**

Right now as you read this there is an excellent chance that you have between three and fifteen pounds of undigested fecal matter stuck in your colon. This waste matter is highly toxic, suppressing your immune system, potentially causing gas, bloating and constipation, dramatically reducing the assimilation of nutrients, and slowing your metabolism. Getting a series of fifteen colonics over a thirty-day period is one of the most important first steps in cleansing and detoxifying your body. Most people lose between three and fifteen pounds simply by doing this procedure. Your hair, skin, and nails begin to radiate and glow with health. Your energy levels can skyrocket, depression, stress, anxiety and fatigue usually are dramatically reduced or eliminated. Food cravings are reduced or vanish completely.

24. **Sweat**

Your body is supposed to sweat. It is a very natural way to eliminate toxins. If you don't sweat, toxins build up in the system. The best way to sweat is in a dry sauna.

25. **Get a chiropractic adjustment**

Every chiropractor uses slightly different techniques. Some are great, some are good, and some not so good. If you have never gotten a chiropractic adjustment, you need one. Because of our lifestyle, our spines get misaligned. Realigning the spine allows energy to flow throughout the entire body. I personally see a chiropractor at least once a month for a tune-up. Even if you have no pain, go to a chiropractor and get an adjustment. See if there is an introductory lecture or ask a chiropractor in your area for some literature that you can read. The adjustments are painless and most people feel absolutely energized after an adjustment. I personally get treated by several different chiropractors because each one has their own personal style and variations on the treatment.

26. Get something to neutralize electromagnetic chaos

As I mentioned, we are being bombarded by electromagnetic energy from hundreds of sources, including satellites, high-tension power lines, computers, cell phones, global positioning systems in our cars, wireless telephones, remote controls, high-definition TVs, etc. We can not eliminate the electromagnetic energy around us, we can only do things to neutralize the negative effects. There are devices which I believe neutralize these negative energies. Some can be put in your home or office and neutralize all the negative energy in the space around you; others can be carried in your purse or pocket, or worn as a pendant. Because of the censorship imposed by our government, it is forbidden for me to tell you the products that I personally use. However, go to www.naturalcures.com, and in the private member area you can e-mail me and I will tell you what I use and where to obtain them. They are inexpensive and work brilliantly.

27. Eat raw organic nuts and seeds

Raw means uncooked. Stay away from roasted and salted nuts and seeds. Ideally, buy them in the shell, they retain more nutrients. There is tremendous life force in nuts and seeds. They are great to snack on throughout the day.

28. Drink no diet sodas

Diet sodas have been called the "new crack" because they are so addicting. Diet sodas will actually make you gain weight as well as make you depressed. Because of the artificial sweeteners used, such as aspartame, they are also giving you a variety of medical symptoms. If you want a soda, ideally, get an organic soda from your health food store; or if you must indulge, drink a regular soda. If you were to stop drinking all diet sodas and replace them with regular soda, you would in fact lose weight. The idea that diet sodas have less calories, thus are good for weight control, is a lie. The exact opposite is true. Remember, all carbonated drinks block calcium absorption.

29. **See an herbalist**

Like all healthcare practitioners, there are individuals who are excellent and whose therapy will give you tremendous, vast and profound results. Seeing a highly-recommended herbalist allows you to be treated in a natural way where you avoid the dangers of drugs. If you have never had a consultation with an herbalist at least once, you have no idea what you are missing. When you take recommended herbs in a specific recommended dosage that is customized specifically for you, the physical benefits that you can receive are enormous.

30. **See a homeopathic practitioner**

Homeopathy is a form of medical treatment that gently brings the body into balance and can cure physical problems. A good homeopathic doctor does not treat symptoms, but he treats the whole person. Highly recommended.

31. **Walk**

People in America are exercising more than ever before, but the amount of walking has dramatically decreased. People in most foreign countries walk between ten and 100 times more than Americans. The body is designed to walk. Walking outside reduces stress, stimulates the lymphatic system, promotes a thin, lean body, and walking and looking at the world eliminates depression and dramatically reduces stress.

32. **Do Chi Kung**

Chi Kung is similar to tai chi in that it is a series of movements that stimulate strength, energy flow, increased energy and many other health benefits. There is a man from Tennessee who is in his sixties. He has the body and skin of an athlete in his thirties. No one would ever guess this man's age. He practices most of the concepts described in this book. One of the things he does, which he believes is a major cause of his youthful appearance and incredible health, is chi kung ten minutes a day. Because the earth's magnetic energy is so much lower today than it was thousands of years ago, he does the simple movements standing on very powerful magnets. This technique is very effective. Practitioners usually feel a major increase in physical energy within just a few days. Sleeping is improved and people report an increased sense of calmness and wellbeing. This course is available on videotape. For more information, go to www.naturalcures.com.

33. **Eliminate aspartame and monosodium glutamate**

Aspartame goes by NutraSweet®. Both aspartame and MSG are classified as excitotoxins. There are three great books on this subject. *Aspartame, Is it Safe?* was written by a medical doctor. Based on hundreds of case studies, the doctor concludes that aspartame is responsible for many distressing medical problems, ranging from headaches and memory loss to hyperactivity in children and seizure disorders. Next, the book *Excitotoxins, The Taste That Kills,* also written by a medical doctor, examines how monosodium glutamate, aspartame and similar substances cause harm to the brain and nervous system, and how these substances can cause Alzheimer's, Lou Gherig's disease, depression, MS, and more. Lastly, *In Bad Taste, The MSG Complex,* again written by a medical doctor, explains how MSG is a major cause of treatable and preventable illnesses such as headaches, asthma, epilepsy, heart irregularities, depression, and attention deficit/hyperactivity disorder.

34. **Do not eat any artificial sweeteners**

Artificial sweeteners are man-made chemicals. They are poisons and should never be consumed. They cause all kinds of health problems. Use raw organic honey, organic raw evaporated sugarcane juice, or the herb stevia. All are excellent choices for sweeteners. Remember, science is not better than nature.

35. **Get an oxygen water cooler**

For a variety of reasons, your body is deficient in oxygen. Increasing the amount of oxygen in the body to the level where it should be alkalizes the body and creates an environment where disease can not exist. One of the best ways to add oxygen into the body is through water. Do not buy oxygenated water at the store. The oxygen dissipates rapidly and by the time it gets to the store, and you buy it, any oxygen that was added is probably gone. I have a water cooler in my house and my offices that adds the oxygen when the water is dispensed. Most people feel an immediate rush of energy and increased vitality. For information on where to get yours, go to www.naturalcures.com.

36. Breathe

Your lungs need to be used. Due to stress levels, most Americans breathe from high up in their chests. If you watch a baby breathe naturally you will notice that they breathe fully and deeply. Their stomach and diaphragm expand as well as their entire chest and back. Deep breathing every day stimulates the immune system, increases metabolism, reduces stress, and brings vital oxygen into the body. Most people are oxygen deficient. Increasing oxygen to the cells can eliminate a multitude of diseases. Cancer, for example, can not live in an oxygen rich environment.

37. Do not eat anything that comes out of a microwave oven

Throw your microwave away. I believe that when you microwave anything it becomes energetically toxic to the body. Eating microwaved food on a regular basis (this includes food that is being reheated in the microwave) weakens your immune system and causes depression and anxiety. Parents who microwave baby formula are poisoning their children unknowingly. The baby formula itself is poison; by microwaving it, it becomes even more toxic.

38. Take digestive enzymes

One of the main causes of indigestion, heartburn, gas, bloating, and constipation is a lack of digestive enzymes in your stomach and intestine. Because of antibiotics, other nonprescription and prescription drugs, chlorinated and fluoride-full water, it has been shown that most people simply do not have enough digestive enzymes in their system, slowing a person's metabolism and blocking the absorption of nutrients. Your body's ability to produce digestive enzymes has been dramatically reduced. Therefore, I believe you need to take digestive enzymes for a period of time until your body is cleansed and rejuvenated, so it can produce the correct amount on its own. Taking digestive enzymes can eliminate acid reflux, heartburn, indigestion, gas, bloating, and constipation. There are many brands available containing a variety of ingredients. Go to your local health food store and inquire as to their recommendations. I give you my recommendations at www.naturalcures.com. It is interesting to note that the majority of people who start taking digestive enzymes lose between five and ten pounds in the first thirty days.

39. **Don't eat in fast food restaurants**

Read the book *Fast Food Nation*. After you have finished throwing up, be glad that you are hearing the truth now. Fast food is simply some of the most nutritionally deficient and chemically loaded "food" on the planet. If the definition of food was "fuel for the body that also encourages life," fast food could no longer be called food. It should be called "fast, good tasting poison," which is a more accurate description of what it is. Oh, and did I tell you that it's designed to increase your appetite, make you physically addicted, and purposely constructed to make you obese? If you eat fifteen meals per week in a fast food restaurant, you have a 90 percent chance of getting cancer or heart disease. Avoid fast food at all costs.

40. **Eat only "organic" food**

You want to eat food that has not been grown with chemical fertilizers, pesticides, or herbicides. Organic food has no chemical poison residue and has much higher amounts of nutrients.

41. **Eat no high fructose corn syrup**

If you look at the ingredients of the product you are buying and see sugar as the number one ingredient, you may be concerned. In order to avoid this, food manufacturers use a variety of sweeteners such as sugar, dextrose, fructose, corn syrup solids, corn syrup, high fructose, corn syrup, multidextrin, and a variety of others. If you were to add up all of the sugars, in most cases sugar would be the number one ingredient in most of these kinds of products. High fructose corn syrup is used primarily for two reasons. First, it is very inexpensive. Secondly, it makes you fatter than the other sweeteners that could be used. The food industry wants you to be fat. Fat people eat more food, thus increasing sales and profits for the food companies. The food industry has lobbied against the public campaign "eat less, exercise more" because they do not want people to be encouraged to eat less. Doing so would decrease sales and profits. Shocking, but true.

42. Do not eat homogenized and pasteurized dairy products

All dairy products are not created equal. Today's milk, cheeses, and other dairy products are radically different in nutritional value and chemical composition than they were fifty years ago. American dairy products are also vastly different than dairy products in other countries. Have you ever noticed that butter from France tastes different from butter from America? Have you noticed that the same kind of cheese tastes different depending on what part of the country or world in which it was produced?

There are vast differences in dairy products due to multiple factors. These differences mean that the dairy products affect the body in vastly different ways. Example: raw milk that has not been pasteurized or homogenized, that came from a cow that was organically raised, was free-roaming, grass fed, and not given antibiotic or growth hormone injections, will affect the body much differently than milk coming from a genetically modified cow that has been given antibiotic and growth hormone injections, never allowed to roam, is fed chemically laced growth enhancing feed, and has been pasteurized and homogenized. The problem occurs when studies are conducted and researchers do not use raw organic milk. They use the chemically laced, pasteurized and homogenized milk. If they were to conduct the studies comparing organic raw milk versus the supermarket variety, we would see dramatically different results. The bottom line here is the standard supermarket variety of milk and dairy products are very unhealthy. Homogenization makes the dairy products scar the arteries in your body and is a leading cause of heart disease. Organic raw, unpasteurized, unhomogenized milk, cheese and dairy products are incredibly healthy. Remember, science is not better than nature. When man gets involved and changes things from its natural state to increase profits, the food no longer is "real"; it becomes a man-made look-alike imitation.

43. **Do not eat hydrogenated oil**

This is classified as a trans fat. Hydrogenated oils are man-made products. They are toxic poisons. More importantly, they attack the artery walls and cause heart disease. They also attack the liver, spleen, intestine, kidneys and gallbladder, causing the internal organs to operate much less efficiently. The bad news is that hydrogenated oil is in virtually every product you buy! The good news is that if you shop at a health food or whole food store, and if you read the labels, you can find many of the products you buy now without hydrogenated oil. This is a good example of how medical science says something is bad, and then later reverses their position. For years heart patients were told to stay away from butter because it was bad for your heart. Instead, they were told to use margarine. Unfortunately, most all margarines are 100 percent hydrogenated oil. Margarines are man-made unnatural products that are deadly poison to the body. Now we hear from the same doctors and medical community that margarine is, in fact, much worse than butter. Stay away from hydrogenated oils and trans fats at all costs.

44. **Speak powerful words**

45. **If you can't eat it, don't put it on your skin**

Your skin is the largest organ in the body. Whatever you put on your skin goes into the body. Many of the things we put on our skin from antiperspirant, moisturizing lotions, cosmetics, insect repellent, sunscreen and perfume are so poisonous that if you put it in your mouth you would die within minutes. I know for many of you this is unrealistic. Remember that I said that if you can't do something 100 percent, do the best you can. If you can't eliminate everything at least reduce the amount of poison you put on your skin.

46. **Don't eat anything in a box, can, jar or package**

Wow! This is a tough one. If it comes in any massed produced packaging, that means it came from a mass production processing plant. If you have ever been in a mass production food processing facility, you would understand what I am talking about. Remember that there are over 15,000 chemicals that are routinely put into the food in the processing cycle that do not have to be listed on the label. Even if you read the ingredient list on the package, there is an excellent chance that the food itself has been produced with chemicals and chemicals have been added. So, virtually all food that you buy at the supermarket that comes in a package is loaded with dangerous chemicals. Secondly, the mass production processing dramatically changes the energetic structure of the food, as proven with the use of Kirlian photography.

Mass produced food in packages is simply unhealthy. Please do not believe what the fancy packaging says. The food companies are only interested in profits and getting you to buy the food. They are allowed to lie, deceive, and mislead so that they can coerce you to buy their product. If you must buy something in a box, jar, can, or package, buy something that was produced by hand in a very small facility. Also look for the words "organic" and read the ingredient list. It still may not be great, but at least it's better than buying mass produced, non-organic products. Do not be deceived by the words "all-natural," "fat free," "sugar free," "low in carbs," "light," "healthy," etc. The food industry has lobbied Congress to allow these words to be put on virtually anything. They are meaningless, deceptive and, in my opinion, fraudulent.

47. Stretch

If your body is supple and flexible, energy easily flows and blockages do not occur. When energy flows it is hard for illness and disease to take hold and manifest. I recommend doing a yoga class, or Pilates, martial arts, or any other kind of stretching on a regular basis. Every morning I spend fifteen minutes stretching. Throughout the day, during my normal activities, I spend a moment to stretch. It feels so good.

48. Get an air purifier

The air in your house is most assuredly not pure and clean. You live, work, and sleep in an environment where the air is flat-out unhealthy. I absolutely recommend an air purifier for your home, your work space and, most importantly, your bedroom. Since you are breathing all night long, it would be a good idea to be breathing the cleanest, purest air you can. Your work space is the second most important. There are hundreds of various types of air filters and air purifiers on the market. I believe some are much better than others. Some are so good that they can also eliminate all the black mold that is causing illness in many homes today. Go to my website, www.naturalcures.com, and in the private members area you can e-mail me for my specific recommendations.

49. **Do not eat farm raised fish**

Companies produce farm raised fish to make a profit. Farm raised fish are given unnatural feed and can be highly toxic compared to their natural wild counterparts. Stay away from any fish that has been farm raised.

50. **Do not eat pork**

Remember, you are what you eat. Pork is a highly toxic diseased food. A pig eats anything in its path, including its own feces. Whatever it eats turns to meat on its bones in a few hours. All pork products are laced with disease and viruses. It is toxic and unhealthy. The human body virtually goes into toxic shock by consuming pork. Massive amounts of blood and energy go to the stomach and intestines to help breakdown and digest this toxic material. Pork is never fully digested in the human body; however, the human digestive system works nonstop in overdrive for up to eighteen hours attempting to neutralize and digest pork. If you didn't eat pork for thirty days and then had some, there is an excellent chance you would be violently ill. Eliminating pork, or at least reducing it dramatically, can have a profound impact on your health and sense of wellbeing. Try and see.

51. **Do not eat shellfish**

More people are allergic to shellfish than any other food on the planet. More people get sick from eating shellfish than any other food. More people die from eating shellfish than any other food.

Any fish that does not have scales and fins should be avoided. This includes clams, muscles, shrimp, lobster, crab, squid, eel, catfish, shark, etc. The fish must have scales **and** fins. Catfish, for example, has fins but no scales. It is interesting that this is one of the kosher dietary laws. Today, we know that fish with scales and fins do not absorb the toxins in the water as readily as sea creatures that do not have both scales and fins.

I grew up in the Boston area. I loved my shellfish more than any other seafood. Occasionally, an algae in the water called the "red tide" would infest the local shores. When this occurred, warnings went out not to eat any shellfish, for doing so could cause sickness and death. However, you could eat the haddock, mackerel, or flounder. You see the fish that had scales and fins did not absorb the poisons into its edible flesh; however, shellfish or any fish that did not have both scales and fins would absorb the toxins and could cause sickness and death. All sea creatures that do not have scales and fins are loaded with toxins and should be avoided.

52. Use a gentle wind project instrument

Our energy fields get damaged due to traumas in our life, all the unnatural man-made electromagnetic frequencies that are bombarding us, and toxic material we put in our body. This energy field needs to be repaired and balanced, and then maintained on a regular basis. The Gentle Wind Project produces healing instruments that are believed to repair and positively influence this field. Although these healing instruments are expensive, you may use one for free. The best part is it takes only five minutes and all you do is hold the instrument in your hand. Go to www.gentlewind-project.org for more information.

53. Do not use sun block

This is one of the greatest frauds in history. The sun does not cause cancer. Sun block has been shown to cause cancer. The ingredients in sun block are now strongly believed to be the number one cause of skin cancer. There is no skin cancer in Africa. People stay in the sun all day long with no sunscreen. It is not the pigment in the skin, as some suggest. People with African heritage living in America have the highest rate of skin cancer, and they stay in the sun the least. You don't want to get a sun burn, so wear a hat or cover your body with light clothing. The sun is healthy for you and the sun should be on your skin. Statistics show that the people who use the most amounts of sun block have the highest skin cancer rates. This goes for tanning lotions as well. Remember, whatever you put on your skin is going in your body. If you can't eat it, don't put it on your skin.

54. **Do not eat white processed flour**

White processed flour is similar to white sugar. It comes from grain that has been chemically treated in the growing process, stripped of all its natural fiber and nutrients, and chemically bleached to make it a pretty white. White flour mixed with water makes paste. You use it to make paper mache. It turns hard as a rock. That's what happens when you eat it. It is an unnatural product that the body does not know how to digest. It has little nutritional value, no life force, and spikes your insulin and causes constipation. Use organic whole wheat flour that has been minimally processed, or buy organic wheat and grind it yourself.

55. **Listen to de-stressing music CDs**

Music has a powerful effect on the physiology. There are several CDs that have been developed that produce stunning health benefits. In just five minutes the music can turn the body from acid to alkaline, relieve tremendous amounts of stress, relax muscles, and provide a tremendous feeling of well being. These can be listened to any time and are perfect for an afternoon five to fifteen minute relaxation and recharging session. For my recommendations, go to www.naturalcures.com

56. **Do not use antiperspirants or deodorants**

Antiperspirants and deodorants contain deadly poisons, most notably aluminum. These poisons are being put on the skin close to the lymph nodes. Anything absorbed in the skin from the armpit gets picked up by the lymph system and first travels to the breasts. I believe one of the major causes of breast cancer in women is the use of these poisonous products. A healthy person should not have an offending odor; however, if you must use an antiperspirant or deodorant, there are all-natural products available. Go to your local health food store and inquire. Don't be misled by the label. Read the ingredients. If you can't pronounce the words, don't buy it. Remember, if you can't eat it, don't put it on your skin.

57. **Do not eat white processed sugar**

Sugar cane, when grown organically, pressed, and dried, creates pure, unprocessed living sugar. You can purchase this in health food stores. It is healthy and good for you. White table sugar, however, is grown with dangerous chemicals, processed, stripped of all its nutritional value and heated, destroying any living vitality that it had. White sugar is a product that has such powerful adverse affects on the body it could be classified as a drug. Real, unprocessed, raw, evaporated cane juice, which is real sugar, is good for you. White sugar is poison. The chemicals used in the growing of sugar cane are known to cause cancer in sea turtles. Those poisonous chemicals used in the growing still remain in the product you buy in the store.

58. **Eat nothing that says "fat free" on the label**

Food companies want you to buy their products. Whatever the hot button is at the time will determine what their marketing people decide goes on the label. "Fat free" does not mean "healthy." When you see "fat free" on the label, be assured that the company is trying to deceive you, so don't buy it. Most fat free products are simply loaded with unbelievable amounts of sugar.

59. **Eat nothing that says "sugar free" on the label**

It if says sugar free on the label there is a good chance the product is laced with artificial sweeteners. Don't buy it.

60. **Eat nothing that says "low carbs" or "net carbs" on the label**

This is the current hot button. The biggest scam going now is the term "net carbs." Manufacturers load up these products with chemicals and artificial sweeteners that they claim have negligible results on insulin levels, so they do not count these real carbohydrates in the net carb number. A product that says it has two net carbs could have as many as forty grams of real carbohydrates. Do not buy these products, as you know that the manufacturers are simply trying to take advantage of the current fad to sell you their products.

61. Do not eat "food bars"

Food bars are man-made products filled with chemicals to provide, first and foremost, good taste. They are highly processed and should be avoided. There are a few all-raw organic food bars. Check at your local health food store and read the ingredient list.

62. Do not eat diet or protein shakes

Like food bars, these are produced by companies whose goal is to make them taste great using the cheapest ingredients possible. With rare exception they should be avoided at all costs.

63. Use organic sea salt

Regular table salt is poison. Sea salt is infinitely better for you. This one small change can also make you lose between five and ten pounds in the first thirty days.

64. Stay away from hot tubs, steam rooms and swimming pools

Swimming pools and hot tubs are filled with water that is loaded to excess with chlorine. Chlorine is a deadly poisonous chemical. People think swimming in a pool or relaxing in a hot tub is healthy. The exact opposite is true. It suppresses your immune system, dries your skin, and loads your body with high amounts of chlorine, scarring the arteries and leading to heart disease. The steam pouring into the steam room is from regular tap water that is loaded with toxic poisons and contaminants. A steam room is, in fact, a poisonous gas chamber and incredibly unhealthy. Swimming is excellent in the ocean or a lake. If you have a pool or hot tub, inquire about a filtration system where no chlorine or chemicals are used. The system that I use employs ozone and oxygen to purify the water. No chlorine or chemicals are put into my pool or hot tub. I have had the water tested, and it was found to be some of the purest water that the laboratory has ever seen. If you can't drink the water, don't swim in it. Some people may say you can't drink lake water or ocean water, and that is true. Those waters, however, are living, fully-vitalized natural waters. Chlorinated swimming pools are something not found in nature.

65. Stay away from psychiatrists and psychologists

Psychiatrists and psychologists do not help the people they treat. Statistics show that the majority of people who are treated by psychiatrists and psychologists actually get worse! Psychiatrists almost always prescribe drugs to their patients. These drugs are some of the most dangerous and deadly pharmaceuticals available today. Did you know that in the last ten years, virtually every violent act committed in schools was perpetrated by a person who either had taken or was currently taking a psychiatric drug. Finally, the research has become so compelling that there are warnings saying that certain psychiatric drugs actually increase the propensity to commit suicide. This is such an important issue that I encourage you to read *Psychiatry: The Ultimate Betrayal,* and if you are still not convinced that psychiatrists and psychologists should be avoided at all costs, I will personally make a donation to the charity of your choice.

66. Do dianetics/scientology

I have been exposed to virtually every self-help procedure known. In many cases, I was personally worked on by the developers themselves. In my opinion the simplest, most complete and effective system of eliminating psychosomatic illness, traumas, and emotional issues is the procedure of Dianetics and Scientology auditing.

67. Stay away from electric tumble dryers

These devices produce massive amounts of positive ions. Positive ions suppress the immune system, make you fatigued, and can cause depression and anxiety. Do this experiment: Go to a laundromat and sit in front of all the tumble dryers in operation, and notice how you feel after just thirty minutes. Then notice how you feel for the rest of the day. Compare this to taking a walk on the beach, near running water, or through an area with lots of trees. These conditions produce life-enhancing negative ions. The comparison in how you will feel can be absolutely dramatic. The clothes that come out of the tumble dryer are also charged with these ions that have negative effects on your emotions and physiology. You will actually feel better if you wear clothes that have been line dried in fresh air.

68. Fast

For my personal recommendations on the best fasts, go to www.naturalcures.com.

69. Don't eat late

It is best to stop eating at 7:00 PM.

70. Smile

There are more muscles concentrated in your face than in any other part of the body. The physical act of smiling strengthens the immune system and releases endorphins from the brain, making you feel better. The act of smiling also changes your energetic field, as evidenced by Kirlian photography. Make it a habit to notice if you are smiling or not. Smile for no reason and do it often.

71. Get and give hugs

Human contact is necessary for life. Babies who are given all the nutrition they need but receive no physical contact grow less, cry more, and come down with all types of illness and disease. In some cases they border on death. Our immune systems are strengthened when we physically hug another human being. Ask yourself how many hugs you gave and got yesterday. You should be hugging every day as often as possible! I am lucky; coming from an Italian home, we hugged and kissed everyone. It is a good habit and provides increased health.

72. Drive less

Driving causes massive amounts of stress. The less you drive, the healthier you could be.

73. Don't use a cell phone and drive at the same time

Driving is stressful enough. When you are talking on a cell phone and driving simultaneously, the amount of physical stress that your body is experiencing can be as much as ten times greater. Avoid this at all costs. When driving, it is ideal to be listening to the correct kind of music, as well as wearing an electromagnetic chaos eliminator to balance out the stressful negative effects you experience in the process of driving.

74. Be thankful

Thoughts are things. Thoughts are powerful. When you wake up in the morning, take a moment and be thankful for the day. Before you eat a meal, take a moment and be thankful for the food. Before you go to bed, reflect and be thankful for the people and experiences you have. Living a life of thankfulness creates happiness, peace and promotes general health.

75. Laugh

Laughing is one of the most powerfully beneficial things you can do. Children laugh, on average, 10,000 times per week. Adults laugh, on average, five times per week. Laughing stimulates the entire immune system, elevates depression and alkalizes the body. In the book *The Anatomy of an Illness,* we hear of the amazing story of a cancer patient who, given six months to live, used laughter to eliminate his cancer! Laugh every day as often as you can even, if you have nothing to laugh about. You will feel better and be healthier.

76. Be lighthearted

There are tens of thousands of people around the world who live into their hundreds. Research has been conducted on these centenarians and has found that the major common denominator is that they take life very lightly. A good motto to live by is "You have to care, but not that much." Instead of being demanding, you would be better off if you had mild preferences.

77. Eliminate florescent lighting

Florescent lighting makes you tired and weakens your immune

system. Get rid of all florescent lighting and replace it with full spectrum lighting. Full spectrum lighting is very similar to natural sunlight, and can have incredible health benefits, the most notable being increased energy and alleviation of depression.

78. **Add living plants in your home**

Real living plants add oxygen to the air, balance the energy in the space, produce life-enhancing negative ions, and are incredibly beneficial to the health of human beings. Fill your house with living plants and flowers. You will feel the difference the moment you do it.

79. **Eliminate air fresheners**

Ideally, don't spray anything in the air; don't use solid air fresheners or the plug-in variety. All you are doing is putting toxic chemicals in the air. It really is insane. In my bathrooms I do have a can of organic citrus oil, which can be purchased at most health food stores. Read the labels. Remember, if you can't eat it don't spray it in the air.

80. **Get a massage**

The benefits of massage are reflected in your:

Circulatory System by:
- helping to develop a stronger heart
- improving oxygen supply to cells
- improving the supply of nutrients to cells
- elimination of metabolic wastes
- decreasing blood pressure
- increasing circulation of lymph

Digestive System by:
- relaxing the abdominal and intestinal muscles
- relieving tension
- stimulating activity of liver and kidneys
- elimination of waste material

Muscular System by:

- relaxing or stimulating muscles
- strengthening muscles and connective tissue
- helping to keep muscles flexible and pliable
- relieving soreness, tension and stiffness

Nervous System by:

- stimulating motor nerve points
- relieving restlessness and insomnia
- promoting a sense of well-being
- relieving pain

Respiratory System by:

- developing respiratory muscles
- draining sluggish lymph nodes

Lymphatic System by:

- cleansing the body of metabolic wastes
- draining sluggish lymph nodes

Integumentary System (the skin) by:

- stimulating blood to better nourish skin
- improving tone and elasticity of skin
- helping to normalize glandular functions

Skeletal System by:

- improving body alignment
- relieving stiff joints
- relieving tired aching feet

There are many kinds of massages. Each masseuse gives a different massage. You may like one and not the other. I get at least one massage a week. They are highly therapeutic, and I recommend you get as many as you can as often as you can. Use different people to experience the full range of treatments.

81. Rest from Friday sundown to Saturday sundown

Each week the moon cycles are in position to promote healing and rejuvenation in the body. Resting during this time promotes the optimal rejuvenation of your cells.

82. Listen to nice music

Certain music has been shown to kill plants and, in humans, dramatically suppress the immune system. Certain music also has been shown to make the body very acidic. Baroque classical music seems to promote the health and vitality in plants, and seems to encourage the same in humans. There are many CDs available whose music has been designed to promote health and even slow and reverse the aging process. Certain music also dramatically reduces stress. Go to www.naturalcures.com for my personal recommendations.

83. Do not take vitamin supplements

Many companies selling vitamins are only doing so to make money. There are many grades of individual vitamins. Most companies use the cheapest grades available. These inexpensive "vitamins" in many cases are chemically produced and are not natural. Most vitamin pills have vitamins and minerals in a proportion never found in nature.

It is true that you are most assuredly deficient in vitamins and minerals. The best way to correct this deficiency is by juicing. The second best way is to take whole food supplements. These are not vitamin and mineral pills. Whole food supplements simply take organically produced vegetables and fruits and concentrate them into a convenient tablet that you can take. When you take a whole food supplement you are getting all the vitamins and minerals in the proportion that nature intended. You are also getting the enzymes and cofactors present in nature. It is interesting to note that many natural plants have up to 30 percent of their composition that defies scientific analysis. That simply means that when you take a whole food supplement not only are you getting vitamins, minerals, enzymes and cofactors in the precise proportion nature intended, you are also getting all of the things that science has not discovered yet. Again, I am forbidden to give you my recommendations here in this book. Go to www.naturalcures.com, e-mail me and I will give you my personal recommendations.

84. **Get out of debt**

Stress is the silent killer. Financial pressure causes a massive increase in stress, which leads to disease. There are several organizations that can assist you in managing, reducing and eliminating your debt. When you free yourself from financial worry you are more likely to be happier and healthier.

85. **Get a pet**

Research indicates that having a pet leads to longer life and less disease. Pets give unconditional love and allow us a non-judgmental being to give love to. The process of being loved and giving love strengthens our immune system, reduces stress, and has a variety of emotional and physical benefits.

86. **Get rolfing**

Rolfing is a specific type of deep-tissue massage technique that releases the fasciae (connective tissues between the muscle and the bone) and dramatically improves posture, balance, and integrates your entire body. Rolfing is generally done once per week for fifteen weeks. Each session is like a very deep-tissue massage and takes approximately an hour and a half. You can find trained Rolfers in your area. Highly, highly, highly recommended.

87. **Get an inversion table**

Machines are available online and in fitness equipment stores that allow you to tilt your body into an inverted position or hang completely upside down. This process is believed to decompress the spine, relieve back pain, increase blood and oxygen to the brain, and potentially slow the aging process. I own one of these machines myself and use it a few times a week. It only takes three minutes and you feel absolutely fantastic. Relieves stress as well.

88. **Get a range of motion machine**

How would you like to get the benefits of thirty minutes of aerobics, forty-five minutes of stretching, and forty-five minutes of strength training in just four minutes? There is a machine called the "range of motion machine" which does just that. Very expensive, but highly recommended.

89. **Do tai chi**

There are many people teaching what they call tai chi. Unfortunately, most tai chi instructors aren't really teaching true tai chi. Tai chi is a series of flowing movements designed to center oneself, relieve stress, increase energy flow, increase flexibility and strength, and promote health and well-being. I have done tai chi for over twenty years and studied with dozens of so-called masters. Not until I learned tai chi from a real Shaolin monk from the Shaolin temple in China did I experience the real thing. The good news is doing any form of tai chi has benefits. If you want to learn the most authentic, most beneficial tai chi, go to www.naturalcures.com for information on videos of the Shaolin monk teaching tai chi.

90. **Use Callahan techniques for urges**

Phobias, stress, uncontrollable urges to eat when you're not hungry, can all be eliminated by using a simple five-minute technique developed by Roger Callahan. His book is called *Tapping the Power Within* and is available by calling 800-931-4721, or going to www.naturalcures.com.

91. **Sleep eight hours**

Ideally, get a full eight hours of solid, deep, restful sleep every night.

92. **Go to bed at approximately 10:00 p.m. and arise at approximately 6:00 a.m.**

In Ayurvedic medicine it is believed that there are cycles that are the most conducive for certain activities. Going to bed at 10:00 p.m. and arising at 6:00 a.m. appears to allow the body to rest the deepest, rejuvenate the most, and gives the person the most energy throughout the day.

93. **Eat organic dark chocolate**

Okay, you need your chocolate. Chocolate is not bad. The ingredients that are put in with the chocolate can be very bad. There are several brands of organic dark chocolate bars that taste wonderful and are filled with real raw organic ingredients. Go to your health food store and inquire. Read the ingredient list. Then indulge and enjoy.

94. **Make your own beer and wine**

If you are going to drink beer and wine, make it yourself with pure organic ingredients. It's fun, it tastes better and it's much healthier for you. Beer and wine are not unhealthy, however, the chemicals on the grapes, the hops, and other ingredients get into the final product. The heat used in processing kills the beneficial living enzymes. It is much better, however, to drink beer or wine than sodas or canned or bottled juice.

95. **Do not use corn oil**

Corn oil is a man-made product. If you took an olive you could squeeze it and you would have oil. But you can't squeeze corn and get oil. Remember, if it is man-made, don't eat it.

96. **Use aromatherapy**

Smells have a powerful effect on our body. Certain smells evoke chemical reactions in the body. Essential oils have many health benefits besides giving a wonderfully pleasant aroma. Inquire at your local health food store into an aromatherapy expert to help you choose the essential oils and aromas that can give you the most benefits.

97. **Commit reckless acts of kindness**

Every day make it a habit to be kind to everyone you meet. The act of showing kindness has been shown to stimulate the body's immune system and give us a greater sense of peace and centeredness. Remember, what goes around comes around.

98. **Wear white**

Colors affect energy. The closer you get to white, the more positive energy you bring into your energetic field. This may not be practical in everyday situations; however, having some white or light colored clothing as your general around-the-house attire can make you feel much better.

99. **Use full spectrum lights**

Florescent lights have negative effects on your body and emotions. The best indoor lighting is called full spectrum lighting. These special light bulbs are very close to natural sunlight. Using these lights can provide reduction of stress, depression, and fatigue while simultaneously increasing energy and positively stimulating the immune system.

100. **Take an afternoon 15-minute break**

Most people wake up to an alarm clock, rush to work, stress, worry and work all day, rush to get home, eat a meal, and sit in front of the television; then they go to bed and prepare to repeat the process again the next day. A fifteen-minute relaxation break, ideally using special music or relaxation CDs, allows the body to decompress, unwind, and rejuvenate. This procedure can increase metabolism, relieve stress, anxiety, tension and depression, allow you to feel more centered, and provide increased amounts of physical energy.

101. **Do not use an alarm clock**

Most people wake to the sound of a loud alarm clock. This shocks the system and starts the body in a stress mode for the day. It is important to awaken slowly and gently. There are alarm clocks that wake you with lovely gentle tones that start off very low in volume and slowly begin to increase in volume. This little change in the way you awaken can have profound effects on your emotions and your body's pH.

102. **Reduce or eliminate air conditioning**

Most general air conditioning is simply not healthy. Air conditioning units as a general rule make the air unnatural, thus unhealthy. Keep in mind that air conditioning did not exist seventy years ago. We think we need air conditioning; certainly, it can make your office and home more tolerable in extremely hot conditions. Use air conditioning less and you will see a decrease in the amount of colds and flus you come down with.

103. Cook

When we create something with our hands we benefit emotionally and physically. When you cook food from scratch you take a much needed mental break, and you can create great tasting, incredibly healthy meals. I personally cook almost every day.

104. Plant a garden

Being in the physical universe, working with living things and creating things with our hands is incredibly beneficial. Working in a garden provides an outdoor environment, exercise, stress reduction, and many more mental, emotional and physical benefits.

105. Don't read the newspaper

You can't fill your mind with negative thoughts and believe that your body pH will stay alkaline. The newspaper is filled with negativity, creating worry and stress. The news printed is almost always misleading, slanted, or in some cases, completely untrue. We hear today of the dozens of journalists who have been found to be fabricating facts for their articles. These journalists, from some of the most well-respected publications, have printed things as news when, in fact, it was completely made up and full of lies. You simply can not trust the newspaper.

106. Don't watch the news

Watching the news fills your mind with negative pictures. My personal studies show that a person's pH can go from a healthy alkaline state, to the cancer-prone acidic state after just thirty minutes of watching a news broadcast.

107. Reduce TV time

The television produces unhealthy electromagnetic energy. High definition televisions produce such powerful negative electromagnetic energy they have wiped out entire computer networks when turned on. The images on TV are negative and stress invoking. But the number one reason I believe you should avoid television is that virtually two-thirds of all the ads you will see are for drugs. When you watch TV, you are allowing yourself to be brainwashed into believing drugs are the answer. Do these ads work? Statistics show that over 90 percent of Americans believe that health is directly related to the amount of drugs you consume. They believe if a parent does not administer drugs to a sick child immediately, they are being a bad parent. These ads are so effective that people who have never seen a doctor are now asking their doctor for specific drugs. Don't think you are immune to the power of these ads. Remember, cigarettes used to be advertised on television. They were proven to be so effective at subconsciously motivating people to buy cigarettes that they were banned.

108. **Have sex**

Sex promotes health.

109. **Eat snacks**

Don't go hungry.

110. **Use foot orthotics**

These promote general health and can eliminate foot, joint, and back pain.

111. **Write down goals**

There you have my basic list of things to do and things to avoid that can bring your body back to a state of normalcy, where disease and illness virtually can not exist. It would be silly for anyone to believe that a person could do all these things all of the time. Ideally, do as many as you can as often as you can. Doing even a little bit is better than none at all. For example, you may not be able to eliminate something 100 percent. At least cut back or reduce, or try eliminating it for a day or two. The more you do these things, and the more often you do them, the healthier and younger you will feel.

CHAPTER 7

Why People Are Fat

If you want to get rich, write a book on how to lose weight. Americans, more than any other people in the world, are obsessed with losing weight. Americans are the fattest people in the world. Statistics vary, but it has been said that over 75 percent of people in America are overweight. This statistic has been rising decade after decade after decade. The interesting thing to note about the fact that we are so overweight in America is that we are doing more to lose weight, yet we continue to get fatter. There are more diet books on how to lose weight than ever before. More people are on diets than ever before. More people eat diet food such as diet sodas, diet prepackaged food, etc. than ever before. More people are concerned about and are eating low fat food than ever before. More people are concerned about and eating low carbohydrate food than ever before. More people are concerned about and are eating low calorie food than ever before. More diet pills and diet aides are used than ever before. More people exercise than ever before. But the fact is, with all this effort being put into losing weight, we are fatter than ever before. How can this be? Keep in mind that this is really an American problem. Although obesity is rising slightly in other countries around the world, America leads the way in people that are overweight and obese.

There is so much data I have on why you are overweight and what you can do to lose weight and keep it off that I could write an entire book about it, and probably will in the future. However, in this chapter

I simply want to give you the basic fundamentals so you can understand why you are overweight and how you've been lied to. In the next chapter I will tell you exactly what you have to do to lose weight once and for all and keep it off forever.

The United States Government, through various agencies, has had a standard party line on the obesity epidemic. As I mentioned earlier in the book, when experts state things they always state them as fact when, in fact, they are simply their opinions. What the federal agencies state as facts as obesity has constantly changed over the years.

Years ago the standard party line was the four standard food groups: meat, dairy, grains, and fruits and vegetables. No one really questioned where the four basic food groups came from, but I saw a poster that was put up in the schools back in the sixties and had noted on the bottom that the poster was, in fact, sponsored by the American Dairy Association. No wonder dairy products had their own exclusive food group. Isn't it surprising that the dairy association, whose only objective is to increase the consumption of dairy products, would strategically put in schools a poster brainwashing kids into believing that in order to be healthy they had to eat dairy products at every single meal? It goes back to "It's all about the money."

The party line for obesity has always been "If you want to lose weight you must eat fewer calories and exercise more." However, there are experts who present information as fact that will tell you that calories are not the issue at all, and you must reduce the amount of fat you consume if you want to lose weight. But there are other experts with just as much scientific proof that claim that fat is not the issue at all; the real culprit is carbohydrates, and if you want to lose weight you must reduce the amount of carbohydrates you consume. Yet another group of experts, with their stacks of scientific documentation, proclaim that food combining is the secret to losing weight and keeping it off forever. However, there is a list of experts lined up, each holding a stack of research documents, scientific proof espousing their fact about losing weight: the glycemic index, insulin secretion, hormonal imbalances, genetics...the list goes on.

As I said in the beginning of the book, no one really knows anything when it comes to medicine, health, disease, illness, sickness or obesity. We all look at studies, general observations, personal experience, anecdotes from other people's lives, and come up with conclusions that we think make the best sense. However, no one really knows why a person is fat or why another person is skinny. Everyone is only presenting a theory. I, too, am going to present my opinion and my theory as to why you're fat, within a system that will allow you to lose weight easier than ever before and keep it off once and for all. I could, as everyone else is doing, present this information as the absolute gospel truth, scientifically proven factual information that is indisputable; however, I am not that arrogant. I'm going to present this information to you, as I always do, with the preface, "Based on the information I have currently, it appears that this makes the most sense. However, as more information becomes available this information may be altered, changed, or 'improved'." With that said, let's look at something we all know is true.

Everyone reading this knows a person who does not exercise; who eats huge amounts of food, including the so-called fattening foods like pizza, pasta, ice cream, cookies, cakes—you name it, they eat it. We all know of a person who falls into this category, yet is as skinny as a rail and never gains a pound. I have a personal experience regarding this. When I grew up my brother could eat anything he wanted, any type of food, any amount, at any time of the day, and he never gained any weight. If I followed my brother and ate the same amount of food that he did, and did exactly the same things he did in terms of exercise, I would have blown up to 300 pounds.

So it appears that some people's bodies are genetically designed to be thin, while other people's bodies are genetically designed to be fatter. At least that is how it appears. However, I was looking through history books about Nazi concentration camps in World War II and I noticed that the people behind the barbed wire, who were in the concentration camps, were all skinny. There weren't any fat people there. I thought to myself, "I wonder if some of those people were genetically disposed to be thin and others were genetically disposed to be fat."

When they came out of the concentration camps and went back to their normal routines, I wondered if some of those people remained thin and other people, because of genetic disposition, got fatter. The point here is it doesn't make a difference what your genetic disposition is, if you're not eating any food for a long period of time, you're going to get skinny as a rail. But that doesn't answer the question about why a person in America has a higher chance of being fat than a person in any other country. Based upon personal experience, thousands of scientific papers, interviews with thousands of people in virtually every state in America over a fifteen-year period, I have come up with some interesting conclusions about why a person in America has a 75 percent chance of being fat.

1. **Most fat people have a low metabolism.**

   What does this mean? This means you can eat some food and even if you eat a small amount your body doesn't burn it off very quickly and, instead, turns it into fat in your body. If you had a really high metabolism you could eat large amounts of food and it wouldn't turn to fat in your body. So the number one reason a person is fat is because of a low metabolism.

   Why is this so specific to America, as opposed to other countries? I will explain. But first, what exactly is metabolism? In simple terms, there are certain organs and glands in the body which regulate how your body burns food for fuel and how it converts food into fat. These include the thyroid, pancreas, liver, stomach, small and large intestines, and colon. When you have a slow metabolism, there is a good chance that some of these organs and glands are not working at optimal levels. Always remember, if you find a problem in the body where the body is not operating as it is supposed to, you have to ask the question, "What caused that not to operate properly?" You always have to look for the cause first. There are many causes for low metabolism, including yo-yo dieting. If you have repeatedly lost weight and gained weight I can tell you that your body metabolism is all screwed up.

   So, let's look at each one of these reasons, and find out what caused the malfunction.

- *Most Fat People Have an Underactive Thyroid.*

  If you have an underactive thyroid, called a hypoactive thyroid, your body's ability to convert food to energy is slow and you have a higher chance of having food that you eat turn to fat in the body. What is number one cause of a hypoactive thyroid? No one knows. Remember, I will always say that no one really knows. I will always say it appears, or it seems, or we believe based on the information we have right now. The answer is really that it appears that one contributing factor to a hypoactive thyroid is the fluoride in the water that you drink. Fluoride is not put in drinking water in other countries. This is one of the reasons why Americans have such a high propensity for an under active thyroid and a low metabolism and being overweight.

  Again, its only one of the contributing factors. There is no one item that is the cause of obesity in America. It is a combination of things, and a number of things that appear to be the reason that we appear to be so fat.

- *Most Fat People Have a Pancreas that Does Not Work Properly.*

  The pancreas secretes insulin. Fat people appear to have a pancreas that secretes insulin at a much faster rate than thin people. A fat person's pancreas also secretes more insulin than that of a thin person. What causes your pancreas to secrete more insulin at a faster rate? The answer: No one really knows. But based on the information that we have, it appears to be some of the food additives that are in the food served in America. Many of these food additives are not put in food in other countries. It also appears that the high amounts of refined sugar cause this pancreas problem as well. American food has more processed sugar than food from other countries.

- *Most Fat People Have a Clogged and Sluggish Liver.*

  The liver is a detoxifying organ. When it's clogged up, your metabolism slows down. What causes the clogging up of the liver? Many of the food additives.

- *Most Fat People Have A Sluggish Digestive System (Stomach, Small And Large Intestine).*

  Overweight people seem to have a problem with supplying digestive enzymes. If you're not producing enough digestive enzymes your food does not get converted as energy and has a higher chance of being stored as fat. What is the reason that you are not producing enough digestive enzymes? It appears to be the food additives that are put in the American food supply. The small and large intestine in overweight people are not as healthy as those of thin people. What is the cause of this? It appears to be a candida yeast overgrowth. Why would you have a candida yeast overgrowth? The reason appears to be antibiotics. If you have ever taken just one antibiotic in your life, that antibiotic killed all of the friendly flora in your intestine and allowed for candida to run rampant, infesting your small and large intestine and colon, permeating the cell walls and slowing down your digestion and elimination.

  So, if we were to ask what is the number one reason for a slow metabolism, the answer is "What you put in your body." The poisons that you put in your body affect your metabolism. These poisons or toxins include nonprescription and prescription drugs, chemical residue used in the growing of food, the artificial food additives used by manufacturers, and the toxins in our water supply, primarily chlorine and fluoride.

  There is another major reason why your metabolism is low. This has to do with exercise. The more muscle you have, the higher your metabolism. Most Americans have an abnormally low amount of muscle in their body. This means you do not burn calories as effectively as you could. The second most important issue in relation to exercise is lack of walking. The human body is designed to walk. An interesting study of thin Europeans, Africans, Chinese, and South Americans shows that the common denominator of thin, lean people is the amount of walking they do on a daily basis. Thin people walk over five miles per day. Americans, on the other hand, walk less than one-tenth of a mile! Lack of walking dramatically reduces a person's metabolic rate.

2. **The majority of people who are overweight eat when they are not hungry.**

   This is caused by two factors: a) stress or emotional eating; or b) physiological food cravings.

   Stress or emotional eating is obviously caused by stress or emotional issues. Physiological food cravings are generally caused by the toxins you put in your body, or candida yeast overgrowth.

3. **Most fat people have a large appetite.**

   If you are overweight statistics show that you find yourself physically hungry a lot of the time. This hunger is generally caused by your body's inability to assimilate nutrients due to lack of digestive enzymes and candida yeast overgrowth. Another reason that you are hungry is that certain common food additives actually increase your hunger.

4. **Most fat people have hormonal imbalances.**

   If you are overweight statistics show that there is a high probability that your body is secreting too much of certain hormones and not enough of others. This imbalance is generally caused by excess toxins in the body or lack of walking.

5. **Most fat people eat larger portions than thin people.**

   This is caused by a combination of factors: larger appetite, inability to assimilate nutrients, physiological cravings, emotion and stress issues, and the food industry's increasing the size of portions. In Europe, for example, candy bars and snack food come in packages that are over 30 percent smaller than American sized portion. Restaurants in Europe serve portions 30 to 40 percent smaller than their American counterparts.

6. **Fat people consume more "diet food."**

   Here is a major mind blower. Most diet food actually makes you fatter. Diet products labeled "diet," "low fat," "sugar free," "low calorie," "lite," "light," "low carbs," "lean," etc., are filled with artificial sweeteners, high amounts of sugars, or chemical additives that actually make you fatter. This is the dirty little secret the food industry does not want you to know. These food additives actually can increase your appetite, make you physically addicted, and cause you to get fatter.

7. **Most fat people are highly toxic.**

Toxins lodge primarily in the colon and fat cells throughout the body. When you are highly toxic your body demands that these toxins be diluted. This causes your body to retain water and increase its fat stores in an attempt to dilute the poisons. This is why you notice people who take lots of drugs become bloated and obese with time.

8. **Most fat people eat before they go to bed.**

When you sleep, your body's metabolism slows dramatically. When you eat late at night the food does not get a chance to burn off and converts to fat easier.

9. **Most fat people are affected by the growth hormone put in meat and dairy products.**

Our meat and dairy supply is loaded with growth hormones. These hormones are given to the animals to speed growth in order to increase production and profits. When you consume meat and dairy you are giving yourself massive amounts of growth hormone. This leads to obesity, and is one of the reasons why children today are maturing earlier and earlier.

10. **Most fat people see themselves as fat.**

Remember Earl Nightingale's discovery he called "The Strangest Secret"? After years of research he discovered you become what you think about. Fat people constantly think about their weight, thus creating the undesired result.

The dirty little secret the food industry doesn't want you to know.

Here I am blowing the whistle on what I believe to be one of the greatest, most devious lies in American history. Remember, "It is always about the money."

The food industry consists of publicly traded corporations. These companies, being publicly traded corporations, have only one objective: to increase profits. The only way that a food company can increase profits is to produce their products at the lowest possible cost and sell those products at the highest possible price, and sell as much of it as they can. That's how they make money. Remember, that's their only objective.

The people that run the food companies, the officers and directors, do not care about the health and well-being of the American public. They only care about the profits. Many of you have a hard time understanding just how greedy these people can be. However, we are now seeing some of these corporate bigwigs being tried and we are amazed at the millions of dollars that they have, and that they will still lie, and cheat, and defraud in order to make more money. Did you know that in prisons around the world there are billionaires. Why? Because the more money you make, the more money you need to make. Making money for many of these people is an addiction. The greed that overwhelms them is unstoppable. Many of these officers and directors are so consumed with making more money they will do anything, and knowingly hurt people, just to make more money. It's sad, but true. Imagine that the executives of food companies think only about how to increase profits, and they need to come up with ways to make their product (food) cheaper. Those ways include genetic engineering and spraying chemical poisons all over the foods, so that the crops won't be damaged by disease or bugs or insects. The soil is loaded with chemicals to make the plants grow faster, or the animals are pumped full of growth hormone to make them grow faster. These companies will do anything to get their products produced less expensively. They also want to sell these products at the highest possible price, and they want to sell massive amounts of these products. So here's what happens.

Food companies will do anything to make their products cheaper. In doing so, the products become highly toxic. If you have ever been in a mass production facility you would be appalled at how food is "made." These food companies also must continue to get you to buy and consume more food. Most food companies have chemical laboratories where thousands of chemical additives are researched and tested. These laboratories are in secret locations and have tighter security than CIA headquarters. The objective is to make the food physically addicting, make the food increase your appetite, and make the food actually cause you to gain weight. Food manufacturers, specifically fast food, are knowingly putting chemicals in the food that increase your appetite, make you physically addicted and make you fatter. Two common additives which appear to do this include the artificial sweetener aspartame, and the sweetener high fructose corn syrup. Like the tobacco industry, the executives of the food industry vehemently deny these allegations. Remember, the tobacco industry denied knowingly making cigarettes physically addicting. The fact is, the American food supply will make you fat no matter what you do. This is why when thin people from other countries come to America, they all seem to gain weight even though they think they are not eating any differently than they had previously.

The food industry is so profit driven that it is lobbying against the national campaign "eat less, exercise more." The food industry does not want people to eat less! The food industry wants you fat and eating more and more food every year.

This is the reason diet products, in the form of pills, powders, food bars, and prepackaged diet foods will never work. The good news is that knowing the truth allows you to take simple easy steps to lose weight faster and easier than ever before. This knowledge also allows you to eat the foods you enjoy, never deprive yourself, and stay thin for life!

CHAPTER 8

How to Lose Weight Effortlessly and Keep It Off Forever

This is not a weight loss book. However, I want to give you the simple steps that will allow you to lose weight faster and easier than ever before, and keep it off once and for all. Space does not permit me to go into the "whys" regarding each step. I can assure you that following these steps will absolutely work. I have struggled with my weight my entire life. I was a fat kid. I tried every diet, every weight loss pill, and even hired a personal trainer, exercising as much as five hours a day. Whatever I lost, I put back on. When I was losing weight I was hungry, tired, and grumpy. I never understood what the problem was; not until I went overseas did I find the answer. While living abroad I ate everything I wanted, yet began to lose weight without even trying. This led me to the discovery of the reasons why Americans are so overweight, and an easy workable solution. Doing these steps will turn your body into a fat-burning furnace and bring your weight to its natural state. These steps also have tremendous health benefits as well.

1. **Drink a glass of water immediately upon arising**

   Ideally, the water should be distilled. Absolutely no tap water. This starts the body's metabolism and cleansing.

2. **Eat a big breakfast**

   It is interesting to note that 80 percent of the people who are overweight eat a small breakfast or none at all. Eighty percent of thin people eat a large breakfast. Your breakfast should consist of as much as you want of the following items. Everything listed should be organic: apples, pears, berries, kiwis, pineapples, grapefruit, plums, peaches, prunes, figs, rye bread, raw butter (raw means not pasteurized and not homogenized), raw milk, plain yogurt (this means no sugar or fruit), wild smoked salmon, beef in any form as long as it's organic, chicken in any form as long as it's organic, lamb in any form as long as it's organic, tuna, sardines, eggs, tomatoes, peppers, salsa, celery, carrots, any vegetable, potatoes in limited amounts, coffee in limited amounts made with pure water (not tap water), with raw milk or cream and raw evaporated sugar cane juice or honey as a sweetener, real tea (not tea in tea bags).

3. **Drink eight glasses of distilled water each day**

   People think drinking water will make them gain weight and be bloated. The exact opposite is true. If you are overweight you need to flush the toxins from your fat cells. Water is absolutely needed for you to lose weight.

4. **Walk for at least one hour, non-stop, per day**

   The body is designed to walk. Research shows that slow, rhythmic movement exercise, such as walking, resets your body's weight set point and creates a thin, lean body. A one-hour walk everyday will change your body dramatically in as little as one month.

5. **Do not eat after six p.m.**

   Do the best you can on this. However, the good news is you can virtually eat like a pig all day long. And if you stop eating after six, you will still lose weight!

6. **Do a candida cleanse**

   If you are overweight, you positively, absolutely have a candida yeast overgrowth, probably throughout your entire body. Losing weight will be hard and slow and keeping it off nearly impossible as long as this condition exists. If you wipe out the excess candida, losing weight will be easier and effortless, and keeping it off will be a breeze. You must get the book *Lifeforce,* which explains the candida cleansing process. Order this book by calling 800-931-4721, or go to www.naturalcures.com.

7. **Do a colon cleanse**

   If you are overweight, I guarantee you that your digestive system is slow and sluggish. Unless you are having two to three bowel movements per day, you are in fact constipated. Cleansing the colon will dramatically increase your metabolism, and you can lose up to ten pounds by simply getting rid of the embedded toxins in your colon. There are many colon cleansing programs available. Inquire at your local health food store for recommendations. For my personal favorite go to www.naturalcures.com.

8. **Eat organic grapefruits all day**

   Remember the grapefruit diet? Well, it appears that there actually is an enzyme in grapefruits that burns fat. Eating grapefruits all day, as many and as often as you desire, will speed the fat burning process.

9. **Absolutely no aspartame or any artificial sweeteners**

   Aspartame, which goes by the name NutraSweet®, will make you fat. All other artificial sweeteners, including saccharin, Splenda® or anything else, should be avoided. If you want the full story, read two books: *Aspartame: Is it Safe?* and *Excitotoxins: The Taste that Kills.* You can order these books by calling 800-931-4721, or by going to www.naturalcures.com.

10. **Absolutely no monosodium glutamate (MSG)**

    MSG is an excitotoxin. It makes you fat, causes all kinds of medical problems, and can affect your mood making you depressed. It also can be physically addicting, like aspartame, and actually make you hungrier. Unfortunately, the food industry has lobbied Congress to pass laws allowing monosodium glutamate to be put in the food and not be listed on the label. There are dozens of words that can be on the label such as spices, artificial flavoring, hydrolyzed vegetable protein, etc., that are in fact MSG in disguise.

    This is why I recommend buying organic food, where everything listed in the ingredient list is something you recognize and can pronounce. Also, MSG is in virtually all fast food, including things you would never imagine, such as pizza. This is why people in foreign countries eat all kinds of food and never get fat. It's not so much the food, but the ingredients used in American food processing.

11. **Take digestive enzymes**

    If you are overweight there is an excellent chance your body is not producing enough digestive enzymes, causing you to gain weight, feel bloated, have gas, indigestion, and constipation. Go to your health food store and inquire. Try several kinds to see which one works best for you. For my personal recommendations, go to www.naturalcures.com.

12. **Absolutely no diet sodas or diet food**

    Diet sodas have been called the "new crack" because they appear to be so physically addicting. They actually make you fat. The reason they are promoted so heavily is because people become physically addicted to them and they are cheaper to make than regular sodas. I did an interesting experiment with people who drank diet sodas on a regular basis. For two weeks they replaced their diet soda with regular high-calorie sugar sweetened soda. Amazingly, no one gained any weight. Even more shocking was 80 percent of the people actually lost weight. One person lost seven pounds! This was stunning to me. Diet foods fall into the same category. Do not eat anything that is being presented as a diet food. They are loaded with ingredients that will actually make you fatter and make you physically addicted.

13. **No fast food or chain restaurants**

    Any restaurant that is a chain or a franchise that sells fast food produces their food in such a way that it will absolutely make you fat. You can actually eat French fries and cheeseburgers and lose weight,—provided that the ingredients that you use are all organic and contain no chemical additives. It is virtually impossible to eat food in a chain or franchise restaurant where the food has not been processed to last for years without spoiling. The food has to be produced as cheaply as possible for the companies to make money. They must add chemicals to make the food taste great and get you physically addicted. This food also has been produced to increase your appetite and make you fatter. Remember, these are businesses whose only objective is to make a profit. If the food tastes amazing, becomes physically addicting, increases your appetite, and makes you fat, the restaurant is assured of success. They are like drug dealers getting their customers hooked on their product. The customer can't get enough and becomes so addicted that they keep coming back for more. This is the sad truth of what is happening in our food industry today.

14. **No high fructose corn syrup**

This sweetener makes you fat and is physically addictive. Just stop buying food at the supermarket, go to a health food store instead. In my personal opinion, do not buy food that is manufactured by large publicly traded companies. Do not buy brand name food. The profit motive is so high you can be assured that it is not good for you. The sweeteners that are used in food produced in a natural way include organic honey, organic molasses, organic fruit juice, organic dates, the herb stevia, evaporated sugar cane juice. Simply read the labels and if you can't pronounce it, don't buy it.

15. **No white sugar or white flour**

White sugar is in fact physically addicting and makes you fat. However, it is still better than any artificial, man-made sweetener. If you want to sweeten something, use the recommendations I listed above. Sugar would be your last option. Artificial sweeteners should not be an option at all.

White flour, as I have mentioned previously, when mixed with water, makes paste. Eating white flour makes you fat; it can also be addicting, and clogs up your digestive system, slowing down your metabolism. Use organic whole grain flours that have not been processed or stripped of the fiber.

16. **Eat organic apples all day**

The old saying is true—an apple a day keeps the doctor away. Apples are loaded with fiber and nutrients; they normalize your blood sugar and decrease your appetite. You should eat at least one apple every day. The more the better.

17. **Eat only organic meat, poultry and fish**

   One of the reasons you are overweight is because of the growth hormone put in meat and poultry. If you want to lose weight, eat as much meat and poultry as you like as long as it is organic, grass fed, ideally kosher, and most importantly, has not been given growth hormone. The fish you eat should not be farm raised.

18. **Limit dairy products**

   If you are going to consume milk, cheese, butter, or any dairy products, eat only organic products that have not been pasteurized or homogenized. The dairy products should be labeled "organic and raw." It may be hard to find raw dairy products in some parts of the country. The next best option is organic, not homogenized, but that has been pasteurized. Your last option is organic that has been both pasteurized and homogenized. Ideally, if you want to lose weight, reduce dairy regardless of what you are getting. Definitely, absolutely, do not consume any dairy products that are not organic because they will have growth hormone in them and slow your weight loss.

19. **Do a liver cleanse**

   If you are overweight your liver is most definitely clogged. Get the book *The Liver Cleansing Diet* by calling 800-931-4721, or go to www.naturalcures.com.

20. **Eat a big, huge salad at lunch and dinner**

   I don't care if your lunch is a cheeseburger, French fries, and a pint of ice cream. Add to it a big, huge salad and eat that first. You'll be amazed how you lose weight. The salad can contain anything you like as long as it is only vegetables, and they are organic. The salad dressing should be organic olive oil and freshly squeezed lemon juice, or organic vinegar. If you really want to speed the weight loss process, use organic apple cider vinegar. Add some organic sea salt, fresh ground pepper or some garlic for taste.

21. **Rebound**

   A rebounder, or mini trampoline, allows you to stimulate and strengthen every cell in the body simultaneously. Gently jumping up and down on a rebounder for just ten minutes a day stimulates the lymphatic system and increases your metabolism. It is very effective for health and weight loss.

22. **Add hot peppers**

Anything spicy or hot will increase your metabolism and make you burn fat quicker. Imagine for breakfast having some scrambled eggs, some lamb chops, and some rye toast with organic butter. Smother the eggs with some organic hot salsa and you will simply lose weight faster.

23. **Use organic apple cider vinegar**

This has some magical property which helps eliminate fat cells from the body. Take a couple of teaspoons before each meal and you will be amazed at how your clothes will become bigger in no time.

24. **Breathe**

Oxygen burns fat. Most people do not breathe enough to stimulate their metabolism and fat burning capabilities. There are several great videos which teach breathing techniques that are simple and quick to do, and that can help you lose weight faster. For more information, go to www.naturalcures.com.

25. **Wear magnetic finger rings**

Special magnet rings worn on the little finger of each hand while you sleep can have amazing results. For more information, go to www.naturalcures.com.

26. **Get 15 colonics in 15 days**

This process will clean your colon, making it easier for your body to assimilate nutrients. This reduces hunger and increases metabolism. Colonics also allow your body to digest food faster so that it will not turn to fat.

27. **Add muscle**

Muscle burns fat. When you add muscle through exercise you are increasing your body's metabolism. The best way to do this is yoga, Pilates, Chinese kung fu, or old fashion basic exercises. There are several videos and books I recommend. Go to www.naturalcures.com for details.

28. **Fast**

This should be number one, but for most people this is the hardest. Going on a proper juice fast for twenty-one days will completely detoxify your body, flush fat cells, and reset your body's weight set point. It is one of the fastest ways to lose weight, and one of the most effective ways to change the body's set point so that you will not gain the weight back. This should be done under supervision depending upon your medical condition. The best book I know is *The Miracle of Juice Fasting*, available by calling 800-931-4721, or go to www.naturalcures.com.

29. **Cheat whenever you want**

You want ice cream, cookies, cakes, chocolate, French fries, pizza, potato chips? Don't deprive yourself. It's better to eat something without guilt than not eat something and feel bad about it. From best to worst, it looks like this: You are offered a piece of chocolate cake. You look at it and decide that you're full and wouldn't really enjoy it, so it does not look that appealing to you. You politely say "no thanks" and feel great about your choice. You feel no depravation. This is ideal. Next would be: You are offered the chocolate cake, and you decide that you want it even though you are trying to lose weight. You say "yes" and eat the cake with happiness and glee. You enjoy and savor every bite. You're amazed at how wonderful it tastes. You are happy that you are experiencing these incredible, pleasurable sensations of this delicious cake. This is not ideal, but it is second best. Next would be a situation where you are offered the chocolate cake and you struggle with the decision. You know you are on a diet, but you can't help but imagine how wonderful this cake would taste. Inside, a voice says that nothing tastes as good as being thin feels. You struggle some more, you really want the cake, but you also want to stick to your diet. You decide to be strong and say "no." This is bad. It is better to eat the cake and enjoy it than not eat the cake and be stressed out over it. Statistics prove that eating food without guilt keeps you thin. Not eating food and being stressed about it can make you fat. Eating food and feeling guilty and bad about it makes you obese.

Lastly: You are offered the chocolate cake and you really want it. But you know you're on a diet and you struggle with the decision whether to indulge or be strong. You feel weak and become upset with yourself because the desire for the cake becomes overwhelming. You breakdown and eat the cake knowing full well that you shouldn't. You feel guilty and bad about yourself. This is the absolute worst. Remember: If you choose to indulge, absolutely enjoy it and be happy. Do not feel guilty or bad about it.

Ideally, if you are going to cheat and want to eat cookies, cakes, ice cream, potato chips, etc., do not buy these products from the supermarket. Go to a health food store and buy the natural organic counterpart. If you like ice cream, you can find all-natural organic ice cream in the health food store. If you want chocolate chip cookies, you can find them in the health food store. The advantage is that if you read the ingredient list and choose wisely, you can enjoy these delicious treats without all the processing and chemicals that make you fat.

30. **Reduce or eliminate the "uncontrollable" urge to eat when you are not hungry**

   Remember, censorship is alive and well in America. The Federal Trade Commission has forbidden me from saying my opinions on how a person can eliminate addictions and uncontrollable urges to eat. And you thought there was free speech in America. If the First Amendment were true, I would be able to state my opinions and conclusions. I can not. However, if you are an emotional eater and have uncontrollable urges and compulsions to eat when you are not hungry, get the book *Tapping The Healer Within: How to Instantly Conquer Fears, Anxieties, and Emotional Distress*. To order call 800-931-4721, or go to www.naturalcures.com.

It's amazing that little things can make a difference. When looking at this list, a good way to attack it is pick one thing on the list and do that for just one day. Then, look for another thing on the list and, while still doing the first thing, add the second thing. Do that until you feel comfortable adding something else. Keep in mind that the items at the top of the list are the most powerful and will create the fastest results. These techniques absolutely work.

It is interesting that people in America don't realize just how fat they are. I was investigating a phenomenon when people were asked to describe their physical build. The options were slender, average, athletic and toned, a few extra pounds, fat, or obese. Amazingly enough, over 50 percent of the people who picked slender were actually overweight. Ninety percent of the people who picked average were overweight. Ninety-five percent of the people who picked athletic and toned were overweight. What this means is that a person may think he has an average build when, in fact, he could be thirty pounds overweight. I had a friend from Australia who was fat. Everyone knew he was fat. He knew he was fat. He said he was fat. Whenever we went out in Australia he was always the fattest person in the room. However, when he traveled to visit Las Vegas a startling observation was made. We were standing in line at a buffet. He looked at all the people in the line, then looked at himself and said, surprisingly, "Hey, all these people are fatter than me."

Americans are fat and getting fatter. Take charge and do what needs to be done. You'll look better, you'll feel better, and you will be healthier. There has been so much positive feedback on these techniques that a book will be coming out shortly to make the implementation of them effortless and painless. For more information, go to www.natural-cures.com.

How to Read Food Labels

Hopefully by now you are convinced that there are many toxic chemicals in the majority of the food that you purchase in supermarkets or eat in primarily chain restaurants and fast food restaurants. Our food supply is different than it was seventy-five years ago, fifty years ago, even twenty-five years ago. Many of you eat the exact same brand of product today as you did twenty or thirty years ago, not knowing that same product is not the same at all. Today that same product could have 100 times more chemical toxins than it did twenty-five or fifty years ago. In an attempt to produce cheaper food, make it last longer, lower costs, make you physically addicted, increase your appetite and make you fat, food manufacturers are loading the food with chemicals and processing systems that only add toxins that destroy any living enzymes in the food, wiping out much of the nutritional value. Food is simply not the same as it was years ago. Today the food is loaded with toxins, depleted of nutritional value, and energetically altered so much that food is, in fact, man-made foreign substances that the body does not know how to handle.

The bottom line is that today it is virtually impossible to go to a supermarket and buy any food that is not full of chemicals, drastically reduced of nutritional value, or energetically altered. It is impossible to go to a chain, franchise or fast food restaurant and get any food that is also not loaded with toxic chemicals, and stripped of nutritional value, making it virtual poison to the system. Ideally, a person would never eat in a chain or fast food or franchise restaurant, and you would never buy anything produced by a mass-production, large food company. But realistically, most people would never do that. Sure, ideally you would buy only organic fruits, vegetables, nuts, seeds, grains, beef, chicken, lamb, eggs, butter, milk, cream, cheese, herbs and spices, and make everything in your house from scratch. Sure, ideally you would eat a majority of live raw food, not cooking it and destroying the natural livings enzymes. But, realistically, most people could never do that.

So is it a lost cause, or is there something you can do to eat food that has much less toxins, much more nutrition, and not been energetically altered? The answer is yes. It may not be perfect, but it will be infinitely better than what you are doing now, and it's simple and easy. I'll give you some rules, and then I'll actually show you how to read the food labels and give you some examples.

The basic rule is when you go shopping, do not go to a supermarket. Major supermarkets are in business to make money. There is virtually nothing in a supermarket that is not loaded with toxins, stripped of nutrition, and altered energetically. When you go shopping for food, go to a farmer's market and buy organic fruits and vegetables, herbs and spices from small independent growers that you can talk to, meet and feel confident that what you are eating is good for you. You can plant your own herb garden or small vegetable garden. Remember, do not use hybrid seeds because that's a nice way of saying "genetically altered by man."

The most convenient way to shop for food is go to your local whole food or natural health food type store. Keep in mind, when you go to a health food store or an all-natural whole food type of store, that not everything in there is perfectly 100 percent okay. Remember, it's always all about the money. These stores, in some cases, are also publicly traded companies that have to make a profit, so you must read the labels. When you go to these kinds of stores, however, you have an excellent chance of finding things that are not loaded with toxins, are packed full of nutrition, and have not been energetically altered, unlike a regular supermarket where you virtually have no chance of finding any food that is not poisonous. The key to reading labels is not to read the front of the package. This is where the company does its advertising. It has its beautiful pictures, its nice names, attractive colors, and all the buzzword phrases that the marketing department has spent millions of dollars researching that will make you think it is healthy and make you buy it. Take the box, or package, or can, or jar, and look for the ingredients. Keep in mind that there can be thousands of ingredients that have been put in this food that, by law, does not have to be listed on the label. The bigger the food manufacturer and the bigger the name brand, the higher chance that it is loaded with chemicals that are not listed. My first general rule: When shopping, don't go to a supermarket. Go to a health food store, a whole food store or a farmer's market.

My second rule is: I never buy anything that is a brand name or produced by large publicly traded food manufacturers. I have been in these plants and I know what it's all about.

My third rule is: I look for small, independent companies from my local area that package food in small batches and make it with loving care. Although these people are in business to make a profit, when meeting them you find their prime motivation is not to get rich or make money. Their prime motivation is to provide an excellent quality product for their community.

My next rule is that I always, always, always, always, always read the ingredient list. I know there are certain things that, if they appear in the ingredient list, I immediately put the box down. Let me give you the most important words you should look for on the ingredient list, and if you see them absolutely do not buy the product.

1. **Anything You Can't Pronounce**

   This is real easy. If you can't pronounce the word, don't buy it, it's a chemical. They can call it anything they want, they can say it's naturally derived, or that it comes from a plant, or that it's all-natural. None of this is true. Keep in mind that food manufacturers lobby Congress through virtual payoffs and bribes to get legislation allowing food manufactures to call chemicals "all-natural ingredients." So the bottom line is, if you can't pronounce it, don't buy it.

2. **Monosodium Glutamate**

   Never buy anything with monosodium glutamate in it. If you're not convinced, read the book *Excitotoxins: The Taste That Kills*. MSG is an excitotoxin. It is dangerous and deadly; it makes you fat, increases your appetite, and causes all types of physical and medical problems.

3. **Aspartame**

   This is also an excitotoxin. It makes you fat, it makes you hungry, it makes you depressed, and it leads to all types of medical conditions, including PMS and migraines. If you're not convinced, read the book *Aspartame: Is it Safe?*

4. **High Fructose Corn Syrup**

   This is highly chemically and physically addicting, and makes you fat.

5. **Hydrogenated Vegetable Oil or Partially Hydrogenated Vegetable Oil or Any Kind of Oil**

   If it's hydrogenated or partially hydrogenated, don't buy it. This is a trans fat. It's deadly, it causes heart disease, makes you fat and causes a whole host of other medical conditions.

6. **Sugar**

   The sugar used in processing is the most refined white powder you can imagine. They have taken natural sugarcane and turned it into a drug. It's put into food because of its sweetness, but also for its chemically addicting qualities. It is also laced with the chemicals used in the growing of sugarcane. This should be avoided at all costs.

   A nutritional comparison between white sugar and whole sugar:

	White Sugar	Whole Sugar
Sucrose	99.6	88 – 91
Glucose	0	2 – 6
Fructose	0	3 – 6
Potassium	3 – 5	600 – 1,000
Magnesium	0	40 – 100
Calcium	10 – 15	80 – 110
Phosphorus	0.3	50 – 100
Vitamin A	0	120 – 1,200
Vitamin B1	0	.023 - .1
Vitamin B2	0	.06 - .15
Vitamin B6	0	.02 - .015
Niacin	0	.03 - .19
Patothenic	0	.34 – 1.18

These comparisons are based on 100 grams. Nutrient amounts will vary due to variations in harvest and growing conditions. This is a comparison not based on just comparing white sugar to whole sugar, but is indicative of the nutritional differences between any processed food and its whole raw counter-parts.

7. **Natural and Artificial Flavors**

If it says natural or artificial flavors on the label, know this is where food industry lobbyists have done a magnificent job allowing the food industry to lie and deceive the public. There are thousands of man-made chemicals that are put into foods to make you hungry, to make you physically addicted, and to make you fat. They are also put into foods to make it last for years without spoiling, and make it so incredibly appealing to the taste buds that you can't stop eating it. Much of the food in today's high-tech processing loses most of its nutritional value, is energetically altered, and virtually tastes like nothing. Food manufacturers then must add chemicals to make the food taste like it's supposed to taste.

Imagine buying an apple, eating it blindfolded and not knowing what fruit it is. Imagine food manufacturers having to inject the apple with chemicals so that the apple actually tastes like an apple again. That is actually happening today. The reason the apple doesn't taste like an apple is because the growers have depleted the soil so much over the years, used so much chemical fertilizers, pesticides, and herbicides, and the food has been irradiated by some of the most powerful electromagnetic energy known to man, that the final product, the apple, no longer has any flavor. Compare this to an organic apple that actually tastes like an apple. Just because it says "natural flavors" doesn't mean it's natural. The food industry has lobbied Congress to pass legislation allowing chemicals that are not natural at all to be called "natural flavors." This is fraud.

However, this is what's going on. Artificial flavors are treated the same way. When you see the word "natural flavors" or "artificial flavors," if you were to ask the food company to individually list the natural and artificial flavors, they would absolutely refuse. My insiders tell me that if they were to list the natural or artificial flavors used, the list could run to hundreds of chemicals put into that food under term "natural flavors" or "artificial flavors." The other major problem with chemical additives in the food is a single chemical may not have major immediate negative effects. But when you combine two or three chemicals together, just like in chemistry class, new chemicals are formed. Scientists at the food companies know this. What these new chemicals do is incredibly dangerous and incredibly powerful—so stay away.

8. **Spices**

This is the other great fraud that the food industry is perpetrating on the American public. Spices sound wonderful and healthy, but they are not. The food industry has lobbied Congress to pass legislation allowing chemicals to be called spices. They are not spices. They are man-made, deadly chemicals, but legally they can be called spices.

When you ask what spices they use, they won't tell you. If it was just organic, all-natural spices, why are they afraid to tell you the two or three different spices they are using? The reason is, they are not using two or three real spices that you may be familiar with. They are using hundreds of chemicals and putting it in the food, but on the label they only have to use the word "spices." So imagine you buy a can of some product and it says "spices" on there. You think they may have put in some basil, some salt, some pepper, some oregano, or something like that. But in fact they have probably put in one or two hundred different man-made chemicals that have been researched diligently in the secret chemical laboratories that the food industry uses to make this food taste like something, and have other desired benefits for the food company. If they don't list individual spices, but just use the generic term "spices," stay away. Also, monosodium glutamate can now be classified as a spice.

9. **Artificial Color**

Any dyes at all, stay away from. They are simply chemical poisons.

10. **Palm Oil**

A deadly oil that is incredibly cheap to manufacture, and causes all types of physical problems.

11. **Dextrose, Sucrose**

These are, in fact, chemically made sweeteners. Stay away.

12. **Sucrulose-Splenda®**

This is one of the newest, hottest man-made chemical sweeteners. In my personal opinion, it is very deadly, poisonous and makes you fat. It was produced so that the food industry could capitalize on the low-carbohydrate craze. Now, products can have "no carbohydrates" or "low carbohydrates" and still taste sweet. The problem is that it's unnatural, it's artificial, and these man-made artificial sweeteners do in fact increase your appetite, make you depressed, cause all types of symptoms (including migraine headaches, PMS, depression, fibromyalgia, allergies), and most importantly, make you fat. So stay away.

13. **Enriched Bleached Wheat Flour, and Enriched Bleached White Flour**

Remember, stripped down white flour or bleached wheat flour has virtually no fiber. It has been totally depleted of all nutritional value and produced in a highly chemical environment, and is actually turned into such a highly refined product that it has many of the same properties as drugs in terms of how the body physically reacts when it is ingested. Really the only kind of flour you want to see is organic wheat flour or organic other types of grain flour, such as rye, millet, etc.

14. **Soy Protein Isolate**

This is a common ingredient in protein shakes and protein or food bars. Stay away from this. You will virtually never see organic soy protein isolate. The reason is that in the processing of soy protein isolate, hexane is often used, which is a petroleum solvent similar to gasoline. Certainly these chemicals, or residues of these chemicals, remain in the food, but they are never listed on the label.

These are the main things to stay away from, but the good rule of thumb is to simply read the label. If the ingredients are not things that you could have in your own kitchen, if the food is something you couldn't make yourself, stay away from it, it's man-made and it is dangerous. In an ideal world you would make your own food from scratch. It tastes better, you don't feel bad after eating it, your energy levels stay high, you don't get depressed or constipated or have gas and bloating.

A good example is ice cream. I have an ice cream maker in my house. I make ice cream every so often for myself, or when I'm having friends over. I buy raw, organic milk and cream made from cows that are grass fed. Remember, raw means the milk and cream have not been pasteurized or homogenized; it has no pesticides or antibiotics, and is incredibly pure and healthy. For a sweetener I use whole organic sugar, which has never been separated or bleached, or I use organic maple syrup. Depending upon the kind of ice cream I'm making, I may use organic vanilla beans, organic strawberries or blueberries, organic chocolate, organic nuts like walnuts, and maybe a pinch of organic sea salt. That's it. One of my favorite ice creams is maple-walnut, and it is also the simplest. I simply follow the recipe and use the milk and cream, a pinch of organic sea salt, organic maple syrup, and some crushed-up organic walnuts. When people eat this they all say it is the best ice cream they have ever eaten. Well, not only is it the best tasting, but it is also the healthiest. People forget how much fun it is for the entire family to spend time in the kitchen adding love to the food that you eat. Buying food already prepackaged and made by major food companies means you are buying food where no love has been added. The energy a person adds to food by preparing it himself actually causes the electrons in the food to spin in different directions, causing a much healthier product for the body.

But I know you don't have time, and you want something that's fast, easy, quick, and convenient. Okay, fine. Go to the store and buy your prepackaged food, but at least go to a health food store or a whole food type store, and please, please, please read the ingredients and make smart choices. It may not be perfect, but it will be infinitely better than what you're doing now. Let me point out just how radically different the food from a regular supermarket is when compared to the exact same kind of food purchased at a local health food store. Keep in mind that these products are almost identical, but the basic differences are these: The food from the health food store will have fewer ingredients, the ingredients will be organic, and there will be virtually no chemicals in the food at all. The food has not been processed so it has not been stripped of all its nutritional value, and it has not been energetically destroyed in the processing plants of the major food producers. The food from the health food store also tastes better because it is made with whole food ingredients. When you eat it you do not feel bad, you do not get constipation, bloating or gas. Most people eat less because of the incredible increase in nutrition and, because it is assimilated into the body so much easier, you don't crave as much. Keep in mind, most food producers want you to crave their food and eat more. That's how they make more money. So the bottom line is, the food from the health food store, generally speaking, will have more nutrition, nothing energetically destroyed, taste better, and have virtually no toxins in it. So let's go through some products and I'll show you side-by-side differences on the labels.

A. **Pancake Syrup**

Health Food Store

Product name: Organic maple syrup

Ingredients: 100 percent raw, unprocessed, unfiltered maple syrup

Supermarket

Product name: Aunt Jemima Original Syrup

Ingredients: Corn syrup, high fructose corn syrup, water, cellulose gum, caramel color, salt, sodium benzoate, ascorbic acid, artificial flavors, natural flavors, sodium pecsametaphosphate

B. **Bread Crumbs**

Health Food Store

Product name: Bread crumbs

Ingredients: Organic wheat

Supermarket

Product name: Progresso Bread Crumbs

flour, water, evaporated cane juice, organic palm oil, sea salt, yeast

Ingredients: Enriched flour, malted barley flour, niacin, ferrous sulfate, diammonium nitrate, riboflavin, folic acid, high fructose corn syrup, corn syrup, hydrogenated vegetable oil, water, yeast, salt, brown sugar, honey, molasses, sugar, wheat gluten, whey, soy flour, whole wheat flour, rye flour, corn flour, oat bran, corn meal, rice flour, potato flour, butter, mono- and diglycerides, sodium, stearyl lactylate, calcium stearyl lactylate, sodium lecithin, calcium carbonate, ammonium sulfate, calcium sulfate, monocalcium phosphate, vinegar, nonfat milk, buttermilk, lactic acid, calcium propionate, potassium sorbate, sesame seeds, salt, parsley flakes, spice, colors, onion powder, natural flavors, garlic, sugar

C. Potato Chips

Health Food Store

Product name: Potato chips

Ingredients: Organic potatoes, organic sunflower oil, sea salt

Supermarket

Product name: Pringles Potato Chips

Ingredients: Dried potatoes, corn oil, cottonseed oil, sunflower oil, yellow corn meal, wheat starch, malto-dextrin, salt, dextrose, whey, buttermilk, dried tomato, dried garlic, partially hydrogenated soybean oil, monosodium glutamate, corn syrup solids, dried onion, sodium casonate, multicacid, spices, annatto extract, modified corn starch, natural flavors, artificial flavors, disodium inosinate, disodium guanylate

D. Mayonnaise

Health Food Store

Product name: Organic mayonnaise

Ingredients: Expeller pressed soybean oil, organic whole eggs, water, organic egg yolks, organic honey, organic white vinegar, sea salt, organic dry mustard, organic lemon juice concentrate

Supermarket

Product name: Miracle Whip Mayonnaise

Ingredients: Water, soybean oil, vinegar, high fructose corn syrup, eggs, sugar, modified food starch, salt, mustard flower, artificial color, potassium sorbate, paprika, spices, natural flavors, dried garlic

E. Salad Dressing

Health Food Store

Product name: Salad dressing

Ingredients: Water, expeller pressed canola oil, balsamic vinegar, vine-ripened dried tomatoes, sea salt, garlic, oregano, basil, parsley, black pepper

Supermarket

Product name: Kraft Fat Free Salad Dressing

Ingredients: Water, tomato paste, high fructose corn syrup, vinegar, corn syrup, water, chopped pickles, modified food starch, salt, maltodextrin, soybean oil, egg yolks, xanthangum, artificial color, mustard flower, potassium sorbate, calcium disodium, EDTA, phosphoric acid, dried onions, guar gum, spices, Vitamin E acetate, lemon juice concentrate, yellow dye #6, natural flavors, oleoresin turmeric, red dye #40, artificial flavors, blue dye #1

F. Granola

Health Food Store

Product name: Granola

Ingredients: Organic rolled oats, organic honey, organic safflower oil, organic sunflower seeds, organic whole wheat flour, organic spiced almonds, organ nonfat dry milk, organic sesame seeds, organic raisins

Supermarket

Product name: Kellogg's Granola

Ingredients: Whole oats, cold grain wheat, brown sugar, corn syrup, raisins, rice, sugar, almonds, partially hydrogenated cottonseed oil, glycerin, modified corn starch, salt, cinnamon, nonfat dry milk, high fructose corn syrup, polyglycerol esters of mono- and diglycerides, malt flavoring, alphatocopherol acetate, nicinamide, zinc oxide, sodium ascorbate, ascorbic acid, reduced iron, guar gum, BHT, cryodypyridoxine hydrochloride, riboflavin, Vitamin A palmetate, folic acid, thiamin hydro-chloride, Vitamin D, Vitamin B_{12}

G. **Sugar**

<u>Health Food Store</u>

Product name: Whole organic sugar

Ingredients: Whole unrefined evaporated cane juice, squeezed dry and ground. Contains the whole dried juice of sugar cane. Dried in its whole state, it is a living food and an excellent source of energy because of the balanced carbohydrates. The molasses is not separated from the sugar streams.

<u>Supermarket</u>

Product name: White sugar

Ingredients: Sugar (Even though the ingredient list from the supermarket simply says "sugar," this is a lie. The food industry has lobbied Congress to allow them to use the word "sugar," when in fact they should say: "Sugar that has been grown chemically, highly processed, using dangerous chemicals, stripped of all its nutritional value, bleached with highly poisonous chemicals to make it look beautifully white and turned into this white crystal powder, which should be classified as a dangerous addictive drug."

H. **Cheese**

<u>Health Food Store</u>

Product name: Raw sharp cheddar cheese

Ingredients: Made with raw milk, produced without hormones, antibiotics, or pesticides, salt, natural enzymes

<u>Supermarket</u>

Product name: Cheddar cheese

Ingredients: Milk, salt, enzymes, yellow dye #6 (Even though the ingredients seem very similar, they are two dramatically different products. There is a huge difference between unpasteurized, unhomogenized organically produced milk used in the organic cheese, and the pasteurized, homogenized milk which is loaded with growth hormones, antibiotics and other chemicals.

I. **Chocolate**

Health Food Store

Product name: Organic chocolate

Ingredients: Organic coca beans, organic evaporated cane juice, organic cacao butter, organic non-genetically modified soy lecithin

Supermarket

Product name: Dark chocolate

Ingredients: Sugar, cocoa butter, cocoa processed with alkali, milk fat lactose, soy lecithin, artificial flavors

J. **Bread**

Health Food Store

Product name: Sprouted whole wheat bread

Ingredients: Sprouted organic whole wheat berries, filtered water, organic dates, wheat gluten, sea salt, organic raisins, pressed yeast, soy-based organic lecithin

Product name: 100 percent rye bread

Ingredients: Organic whole rye flour, water, sourdough culture containing organic whole rye flour and water, sea salt

Supermarket

Product name: Wonder Bread

Ingredients: Flour, barley malt, ferrous sulfate, niacin, thiaminmonotrite, riboflavin, folic acid, water, high fructose corn syrup, yeast, soybean oil, salt, calcium sulfate, wheat gluten, soy flour, sodium stearyl lactylate, calcium dioxide, calcium iodate, diammonium phosphate, dicalcium phosphate, monocalcium phosphate, mono- and diglycerids, ethoxylated mono- and diglycerides, calcium carbonate, datem, yeast nutrients, ammonium sulfate, ammonium chloride, wheat starch enzymes, tricalcium phosphate, calcium propionate

K. Chocolate Chip Cookies

Health Food Store

Product name: Chocolate chip cookies

Ingredients: Organic unbleached flour, organic evaporated cane juice, organic palm shortening, organic chocolate chips, organic brown rice syrup, walnuts, vanilla, nongenetically modified soy lecithin, organic molasses, baking soda, unsweetened cocoa, sea salt

Supermarket

Product name: Chips Ahoy Chocolate Chip Cookies

Ingredients: Wheat flour, niacin, reduced iron, thiamin-monotrate, riboflavin, folic acid, sugar, chocolate dextrose, cocoa butter, soy lecithin, sugar, partially hydrogenated soybean oil, high fructose corn syrup, baking soda, ammonium phosphate, salt, whey, natural flavors, artificial flavors, caramel color

L. Food Bar

Health Food Store

Product name: Food bar

Ingredients: Organic almond butter, organic date paste, organic aguava nectar, organic brown rice protein, organic raisins, organic flax sprouts, organic sesame seeds, organic brown rice crisps

Supermarket

Product name: Marathon Energy Bar

Ingredients: Corn syrup, soy protein isolate, peanut flour, whey protein isolates, calcium caseinate, sugar, cocoa butter, chocolate, lactose, skim milk, milk, milk fat, soy lecithin, artificial flavor, corn syrup, sugar, partially hydrogenated soybean oil, skim milk, milk fat, glycerine, lactose, caramel, salt, artificial flavors, peanuts, rice, oats, brown sugar, sugar, wheat, sugar, salt, barley malt, rice, sugar, salt, barley malt, brown sugar, glycerine, high fructose corn syrup, chocolate, salt, barley malt, Vitamin A, palmatate, tricalcium phosphate, magnesium oxide, ascorbic acid, Vitamin E acetate, niacinimide, D calcium, pantothenate, ferrous funarate, zinc oxide, pyridoxina hgl, riboflavin, thiamin monotrite, folic acid, biotin, cyanocabalamin

Product name: Advantage Atkins Bar

Ingredients: Soy protein isolate, hydrogenised collagen, whey protein isolate, calcium, sodium caseinate, glycerine, polydextros, cocoa butter, cocoa powder, water, natural coconut oil, soy nuggets, soy protein, rice flour, malt, salt, cellulose, olive oil, natural flavors, artificial flavors, lecithin, decaffeinated coffee, multidextrine, guar gum, citric acid, sucrolos, tricalcium phosphate, calcium carbonate, magnesium oxide, Vitamin A, Vitamin C, thiamin, riboflavin, prydoxine cyanocovalamin, Vitamin E acetate, niacin, biotin, pantothenic acid, zinc, folic acid, chromiumkelate, Vitamin K, selenium

M. **Fig Bars**

Health Food Store

Product name: Fig bars

Ingredients: Organic whole wheat flour, organic figs, organic honey, grape or pear juice, canola oil, corn starch, molasses, malt syrup, sea salt, cultured whey, lecithin, baking soda

Supermarket

Product name: Fig Newtons

Ingredients: Wheat flour, niacin, reduced iron, thiamin-monotrate, riboflavin, figs preserved with sculpture dioxide, sugar, corn syrup, high fructose corn syrup, whey, partially hydrogenated soybean oil, maltic acid, salt, baking soda, calcium lactate, yellow corn flour, soy lecithin, potassium sorbate, artificial flavors, malted barley flour

N. **Protein Powder, Shake, or Meal Replacement**

Health Food Store

Product name: Protein powder

Ingredients: 100 percent raw certified organic hemp protein powder

Product name: Meal shake

Ingredients: Organic spuralina, organic blue-green algae, organic chlorella bokensel algae, barley, alfalfa, organic wheat grasses (barley grass, alfalfa grass, wheat grass), organic purple dulse seaweed, organic beetroot, organic spinach leaf, organic rosehips, organic orange and lemon peels

Supermarket

Product name: Slimfast

Ingredients: Sugar, fructose, cocoa processed with alkali, whey protein concentrate, soy protein isolate, gum, arabic cellulose gel, sweet dairy whey, nonfat dry milk, powdered cellulose, guar gum, soybean lecithin, carrageean, dextrox, cellulous gum, soy fiber, modified corn starch, xanthan gum, multidextrin, artificial flavors, aspartame, calcium phosphate, magnesium oxide, calcium carbonate, sodium asorbate, Vitamin E acetate, phericortho phosphate, niacinimide, zinc

Product name: Protein powder

Ingredients: Organic fermented soy protein, skim milk, yogurt powder, honey

oxide, calcium pantophenate, magnesium sulfate, copper glucanate, pridoxine hydrochloride, thiamine mononitrates, Vitamin A palmatate, chromium chloride, riboflavin, biotin, folic acid, sodium molybdate, sodium selenite, phylloquinone, potassium iodine, choletalciferol, cyanocobalamin

I could do a hundred of these, comparing a brand name supermarket product to its almost identical counterpart purchased from a health food store and manufactured by a small independent company. There are huge differences between what is available in standard supermarkets and what is available in health food or whole food type stores. Keep in mind, again, you must read the ingredients yourself. Just because it's in a health food store or a whole food store does not mean it's good. Read the labels. When you purchase wisely, you will be buying products that:

- Have almost no toxins
- Have far more nutrition
- Taste better
- Make you feel better
- Will not give you gas, bloating, headaches, spaceyness, constipation, etc.
- Will not make you hungrier
- Will not make you fat
- Will not get you physically addicted
- And you will be supporting small, independent, and in many cases local people who are trying to produce products that taste great and are good for you.

When you go to your local supermarket and buy name brand products and/or products from major publicly traded food corporations, you are supporting the multinational companies that are hurting local growers and independent farmers, and causing massive amounts of illness and disease; not only in America, but in countries around the world. It is my opinion that these large multinational corporations are exploiting and taking advantage of people through their clever use of advertising, and knowingly giving us food filled with chemicals that increase our appetite, get us physically addicted, and make us fat, all in the name of profit. Remember, I am not being fanatical in telling you to eat only raw uncooked fruits, vegetables, nuts, and seeds. I am saying to take little steps and go at a pace that is right for you.

Many of you simply are unwilling to change any of your eating habits. Some of you like your hotdogs smothered with mustard and ketchup, and nothing is going to change that. That's fine. Eat your hotdog and enjoy it. But instead of buying the buns, the hotdogs, the mustard and ketchup at the supermarket, why don't you get some incredibly delicious hotdog buns from the local health food or whole food store? It will taste better, have no toxins in it, and be packed full of nutrition. Don't buy the brand name hotdogs filled with nitrites and made from diseased animal parts that would make you sick if you saw them being processed. Instead, get an organic nitrite-free hotdog, ideally one made with prime cuts of beef instead of beef parts. Buy some organic mustard and ketchup, and then enjoy your hotdogs.

If you like your snack food, that's fine. Go to the health food store and try various kinds of snack food to munch on; many of them are very sweet and incredibly tasty. Taste will vary, so try different kinds to see which ones you like. As I write these words, I purchased five different sweet snacks at my health food store. The first one has four ingredients: pure raw carob, coconut, pure cane crystals, pure maple syrup. All of the ingredients are organic, have not been cooked, are all raw, and are real living food. They taste incredible. Another one has as its ingredients: raw organic sunflower seeds, raw organic raisins, raw organic bananas, raw organic maple syrup, and fennel. These are sweet and delicious. Another one is this incredible almond brittle made with raw almonds, pure vanilla beans and crystals of pure cane. It's simple, real, all-natural, and toxin free. And here's the great part: Last night, to see how I would feel, I ate this huge bag of this almond brittle all in one sitting. I didn't feel bloated, I didn't get a sugar rush, I didn't have a spike in moods, I felt absolutely fine, and I slept like a baby. If I had done the same thing with some almond or peanut brittle purchased from the store and loaded with chemicals, I would have felt horrible, bloated, gassy and would have tossed and turned all night.

Just remember that name brand products and large multinational publicly traded corporations are investing tens of millions of dollars in research to find out what the hot buttons are to get you to buy their products. Don't believe their slick, deceptive ads, and don't believe what's written on the front of the package. You simply are being deceived. Read the ingredients and remember as you read them that many toxins that were used in the processing of the food are not listed on the ingredients, and many toxins that are actually put in the food do not have to be listed on the ingredients.

It's estimated that over 95 percent of all food purchased has as many as 300 chemicals added to each product that are **not** listed on the label. It's scary, but true. This is the power of the food industry and the lobbyists. If you want to eliminate sickness and disease, if you want to prevent sickness and disease, if you want to be thin, then you must increase the amount of raw uncooked organic food in your diet. The only way you can do this is stay away from the supermarket. So, the general rule of thumb is to do all your shopping at a local farmers market and make sure that all of your fruits, vegetables, herbs, nuts and seeds are 100 percent organic and raw. When purchasing other food products, avoid the supermarket at all costs and buy your food products from your local health food or whole food type store. If the product is manufactured by a large, publicly traded corporation, or is a well-known brand name, avoid it. Lastly and most importantly, whenever you buy anything, read the ingredients.

Restaurants

I am often questioned about eating in restaurants. A restaurant is not a restaurant is not a restaurant. There are vast differences between the kinds of restaurants you go to. I'm not talking about the food, I'm talking about the kind of restaurant. Virtually all restaurants have the following problems:

In order to make a profit they have to buy the cheapest food available. Restaurants get their food primarily from large, bulk food suppliers that supply hundreds of restaurants in a given area. Much of the food you eat in any restaurant has not been cooked at the restaurant; rather, it has simply been finished off or heated up. It gets worse with restaurants that are vast in number, such as franchises, chains and fast food. Most restaurants use microwave ovens to reheat the food right before serving. Most restaurants, like large food manufacturers, use frying oil all day and, in many cases, for days on end. The problem with this is once you heat the oil for frying it goes rancid in a very short period of time. All the food coming out of the rancid oil is highly carcinogenic.

I went into a very nice restaurant and was about to order, but wanted to ask some questions. I love fresh guacamole. I make it at my house with all raw organic ingredients and it is absolutely delicious. I saw they had guacamole on the menu so I inquired, was the guacamole made fresh? The waiter told me yes. I inquired a little further. I asked, "So you actually take avocados and mash them up in the back or does it come in prepackaged mix?" And he said, "Oh, well we do get a mix, but we add water and make it fresh every day." His idea of fresh and homemade and my idea were two different things. You see, this guacamole was not made in the back with fresh avocados, tomatoes, lime juice, onions, etc. Instead, it came as a powdered mix to which water was added. When I asked what the ingredients of the mix were, of course he didn't know. I persuaded him to go and find the package and bring me the ingredient list. There are over three dozen ingredients on the label, including monosodium glutamate.

I asked if the salad was fresh. He thought for a moment and said "No. It actually comes in bags that have been prepackaged." The problem with this, of course, is that in order to retain freshness the "fresh salad" has to be sprayed with chemicals. I asked if the chicken was fresh, or did it come prepackaged and frozen. Not surprisingly, it came prepackaged and frozen. Virtually all the sauces, all the mixes, and all the flavoring agents used came in boxes, cans, or packages. This is the main problem with restaurant food.

So, what do you do? Basically, you can be a fanatic and not eat in any restaurant unless it's an all-natural, totally organic restaurant, or you can simply eat really well at home and stay away from chains, franchises, and food as best you can. When you go to a good quality restaurant, simply ask if you can tour the kitchen and see some of the food being prepared. Most managers welcome this. It will give you a chance to meet the manager and/or the owner and inquire about how the different dishes are made. You can then see which one would be using the highest quality and the freshest ingredients. You can also simply ask to eliminate things. Example: I happen to like fried chicken wings. I make them at home myself, my mother taught me how. We take organic chicken wings, lightly dust them in organic whole wheat flour with sea salt and organic black pepper, and gently fry them in a little bit of extra virgin organic olive oil. They are absolutely delicious. When I go to a restaurant, I know that most chicken wings are purchased pre-made and pre-breaded, and are simply thrown into rancid oil in a fryer in the back, then smothered in a sauce, all of which contain massive amounts of monosodium glutamate. Therefore, I don't eat chicken wings in restaurants. So basically, I ask a few questions and make some intelligent choices. And remember, you have to care, but not THAT much. You have to do what you feel good about and happy about and not be stressed out about your decisions.

I have a close friend who is not only a vegetarian, but eats only raw, uncooked food. She is not stressed out or fanatical about it, that's just what she eats. We went to a restaurant and I ordered some salmon sushi. I know the salmon was caught in the wild, and the rice is made with pure ingredients. I also liked the cucumber and onion salad they make. The fresh ginger and wasabi was also delicious and made fresh at the restaurant. Although the restaurant does not use organic ingredients, it's a matter of degree. My meal could be classified as relatively healthy. Far from ideal, but also far from something you could find in a fast food restaurant. At least there were no hydrogenated oils, monosodium glutamate, aspartame or massive amounts of chemicals. My friend, being a vegetarian and a raw foodist, had limited options, but her attitude about what she wanted was the key. She inquired about her choices and made her selections. We had lovely conversation, and her food was secondary in nature to our discussions. She wasn't stressed, uptight, or fanatical. She wasn't judgmental or pushing her ideas and values upon me. Maybe someday I will eat only raw food too. For right now, I love my organic lamb, chicken, beef and various kinds of cooked food. The point is, knowing all this information doesn't mean you have to do it all in order to receive benefits. Do a little or a lot, based on what you feel good about. Even making some simple modifications and changes to your diet could have dramatic impact.

CHAPTER 10

Not Convinced?

This book is filled with some very basic premises from which our conclusions are built. The most basic is that there are natural nondrug and nonsurgical cures for virtually every disease. There are natural nondrug and nonsurgical ways to prevent you from virtually ever getting sick. Many organizations, including the FDA, the FTC and the pharmaceutical industry, are working diligently to prevent you from hearing or learning about this information. The news media, including newspapers, magazines, television and radio, are biased toward the pharmaceutical industry and present half-truths and outright lies in relation to healthcare. If you're still not persuaded then consider these thought provoking ideas.

1. Still not convinced it's all about the money? Then consider this:

    - It has been reported that corporate corruption is at an all-time high. There is more corporate fraud going on than ever before.

    - Schools get $500 for every student who is on the drug Ritalin. This gives a major incentive for schools to diagnose a child with attention deficit disorder, and demand or require the child be put on the drug.

    - Reality shows are at an all-time high in terms of viewership. The producers make money by helping to create as much pain and misery for the contestants as possible. As one of the biggest producers of reality TV has been quoted as saying "There is appeal in other people's misery." All in the name of money and greed, do these producers victimize the participants of reality TV. In many cases, these contestants leave the show permanently emotionally scarred from their experience. The producers do not care. All they care about is how much money they will make at the expense of other people. It seems very similar to ancient Rome, when people were entertained by watching other human beings being fed to the lions. It is a sad state of affairs that greed seems to be at an all-time high in America.

- Communities make so much money on speeding tickets that the government refuses to put limiters on cars, even though they know that it would save over 100, 000 people a year from death or injury. But it would also cost the oil companies huge profits. They have a law that says you have to wear your seatbelt. Therefore, cars have to have seatbelts installed. There is a law limiting the amount of emissions cars can give; therefore, cars have to put catalytic converters and do things to limit emissions. There is a law that says that you can't, under any circumstances, exceed the national speed limit. Why, then, are cars not required to have limiters so that they don't go that fast? The answer: It would cost the communities huge amounts of money in profits from speeding tickets, and the oil companies enormous profits in gasoline. It would also reduce huge amounts of money spent on car repairs and would save all types of money for individuals on hospital costs, injuries and missed work, as well as save lives.

- E-mail spamming could be stopped instantly. All Congress would have to do is pass a law forbidding credit card companies to process payments from spam e-mail. Any credit card company that processed a payment from a spam e-mail would face severe fines or loss of the right to process any credit cards, or jail. The credit card companies then would take the responsibility of knowing their customers and finding out how business was generated. E-mail spamming would stop. The policing action is simple. All the government has to do is order a product from some spam e-mail and then charge the credit card company with the violation. The reason this is not being done is because the credit card companies make tens of millions of dollars in processing business from spam e-mail. Since they've lobbied Congress, Congress will not pass laws to hurt the companies that are giving them money.

- Self-serve gas stations were set up so that the corporations can make more money.

- When calling a company, many people have experienced not having the phone answered by a person, but rather a voice activated system with several menu options. Many people know that you can call a company and be asked a series of questions about the nature of your call, and if the reason for your call is a specific reason to push 1, if it's another reason push 2, yet another reason push 3. Then when you get there, there is a new list of options, push 1 for this, 2 for this, three for this. Then when you do that, there's yet another list of options; there can be as many as ten different menus you go through. Why is this being done? It's all about the money. It saves the company huge amounts of money knowing that the majority of people will get frustrated and hang up; therefore, they don't have to take the call and spend the money on customer service.

- The pharmaceutical industry focuses more time and money on marketing than on the development of new drugs.

- Donald Trump is reported as saying "All trading done at the highest levels is illegal. It's all insider trading."

- Time Warner reported that banks lie to you in order to make more money, and recently reported that there are ten secrets or ten specific lies that banks tell customers on a regular basis that cost the consumer money and make the bank more profit.

- Newspapers, magazines, television and radio commonly talk badly about all-natural products, while at the same time running ads for products that they are not bashing. This is done purposely. This occurs most blatantly on websites.

- Health food and vitamin companies are being gobbled up and are either owned directly or indirectly by the pharmaceutical industry.

- Many "newsletters" or books promote certain supplements. Most people do not know that the owners of these newsletters or books are the same people that actually sell the supplements. This is misleading and fraudulent, but very profitable for the big corporations. Magazines and newspapers commonly run positive articles on products if those companies commit to large advertising contracts. This is fraud, and it happens virtually all the time. What it means is you can't believe anything you read in magazines and newspapers, because you don't know if the article is really a payoff for the large amounts of advertising the publisher receives.

- Companies routinely shift jobs overseas. The main reason: It has been reported that it is twenty-five times more expensive to hire an American worker compared to his Asian counterpart. Companies are only in business to make money and will continue to shift jobs in production overseas where it is less expensive to produce the goods and services.

2. Not convinced that the FTC and FDA, as well as maybe TV, radio, and news organizations, are suppressing and censoring information? Then consider this.

- CBS refused to air a thirty-second commercial from a group that was critical of the Bush administration. CBS also did not air the mini-series "The Reagans" because of pressure from conservative groups and advertisers.

- I just received an e-mail stating "Print publishers depend on drug companies for a huge part of their advertising, and may be reluctant to take an ad that antagonizes their best customers." All bets are off if the companies themselves actually apply pressure.

- Disney will not distribute a film critical of President Bush because it could jeopardize the massive tax breaks it gets on its Florida theme parks. Remember, President Bush's brother is governor of Florida. It was reported that an industry insider was quoted as saying, "Should this be happening in a free and open society, where the moneyed interests essentially call the shots regarding the information that the public is allowed to see and hear about?"

- The natural supplement ephedra was banned, but the pharmaceutical version, ephedrine, was not banned. The natural version was taken off the market, but the dangerous chemically produced synthetic version is still allowed to be sold. This shows how the FDA protects the pharmaceutical industry.

- The developer of an all-natural diabetes cure was offered $30 million not to market it.

- Many times when you see an alternative healthcare practitioner, they will have you sign a whole host of forms, disclaimers, release forms, and statements asserting that they are not trying to cure or prevent any disease, and that you are seeing them under your own free will. Because of our litigious society, and because of oppression by the government regulating bodies, these wonderful individuals, by risking so much, must take these measures in order to protect their ability to treat people who need their treatment.

- Vaccines are loaded with poisons. Those who get vaccines are more likely to become sick in the short-term and in the long-term than those who do not get vaccines.

3. Still not convinced that the media is biased, deceiving, and lying to you about many topics? Then consider this:

   - Bill O'Reilly has been quoted as saying "The deception going on in the media is appalling."

   - I get approached all the time by newspapers and magazines with offers of writing positive articles about me or any of my products if I commit to advertising in their publications.

- News organizations often create fake stories by putting together groups of people to yell and scream for the cameras, and the minute the cameras get turned off everyone walks away and goes home. Most events you see on television are actually staged by the news organization.

- Numerous journalists have recently been convicted of writing false and fraudulent articles. Journalistic fraud is now becoming commonplace. It is reported that many journalists are being offered financial incentives to write articles that present a certain viewpoint.

- Many news articles are actually written by individuals who are on the payroll of the companies talked about in the article. An example recently was an article with a headline, "Despite known hazards, many potential dangerous dietary supplements continue to be used." This particular article was written by a medical doctor who was on the payroll of the drug industry. It is not news, it is not true, it is not accurate, and it is not unbiased journalism. It is a debunking campaign put out by the pharmaceutical industry to get people away from excellent, safe and effective natural remedies, and to continue to be brainwashed into believing drugs are the only answer for illness and disease.

- Pharmaceutical companies, with the huge amounts of money they have at their disposal, set up and paid for websites by the hundreds debunking natural remedies. Many of these websites are set up, paid for and funded by the pharmaceutical industry, and are domained in foreign countries. Usually, one small group of people actually runs and maintains hundreds of websites, so an individual consumer thinks that there are these independent organizations around the world saying how bad natural remedies are and how good drugs are. This is absolutely not the case. This is propaganda at its most flagrant form.

- The four basic food groups promoted for years was actually invented by, promoted by, and funded by the dairy association. The food pyramid today was put into effect by our government after massive amounts of lobbying by the food industry. The four basic food groups and the food pyramid have nothing to do with health and nutrition, but are designed to brainwash people into eating a certain way for the benefit of the food industry.

- The media hide the truth about the dangers of nonprescription and prescription drugs. There are very few articles written about how lethal over-the-counter nonprescription and prescription drugs really are. However, the number of articles that have been written and broadcast stating the dangers of natural supplements such as herbs, vitamins and minerals is staggering. The fact is drugs, both over-the-counter nonprescription and prescription drugs, are infinitely more dangerous than any vitamin, mineral or herb. There are virtually no reported cases of anyone dying from taking a natural supplement in its proper dose. However, there are hundreds of thousands of documented deaths that have occurred by taking an over-the-counter nonprescription or prescription drug in its proper dosage.

- Through powerful lobbying, the Atkins and the low-carb craze is at an all-time high. I promoted the Atkins diet on television for two years, but after thoroughly researching the workings of the Atkins organization I found it to be riddled with deceptions, lies and fraud. Isn't it interesting that for years no one in the news media promoted the Atkins diet as a healthy, safe way to lose weight? All of a sudden, out of nowhere, everyone is talking about how wonderful the Atkins program is. This is one of the greatest weight loss scams of all time.

4. Still not convinced that right now your body is loaded with toxins causing you all types of illness, disease, depression, stress, and anxiety? Then consider this:

- People who golf come home with massive amounts of chemical fertilizer absorbed in their body from breathing the air and walking the golf course.

- All injections from botox, collagen, insulin and vaccines are loaded with poisonous toxins. Many of these are animal based and are filled with deadly pathogens and chemicals.

- There are so many toxins in our environment and food that even people who live in the most remote parts of the world have been found to have massive amounts of toxins in their fat cells, even though the toxins do not exist in their local environment. This is a toxic world, and no one is immune. You are filled with toxins right now.

- Because of toxicity, most people do not assimilate high amounts of nutrients from what they are eating.

- Toxins make a person deficient in nutrients.

5. Still not convinced that the politicians and various government agencies are out of control and operating un-policed? Then consider this:

- Did you know that there is a law that allows the government to walk up to you on the street and take away any money you have in your pocket, as well as confiscate any property that they want such as your car and home? Did you know that this can be done to any person living in America and you don't even have to be charged with a crime, you don't even have to be arrested? If you want to get your money or personal property back, you then have to file suit against the government and it could take up to two years.

- Did you know that there is a law in America that allows the government to take any person living in America and, without arresting them and without charging them with a crime, take that person and incarcerate them for an unlimited amount of time, as well as forbidding that person from having any contact with any person, including an attorney? This person— who has not been arrested or charged with a crime—can be held and incarcerated, and can be denied all access to the legal system. I know this sounds like the Gestapo in Nazi Germany, but it is absolutely true, and most people just don't realize just how much the U.S. Government is becoming a police state.

- Did you know that Congress makes themselves exempt to virtually every law they pass? It's unbelievable but true. Congress will pass a law requiring handicapped access to all businesses, but makes the government exempt. It will pass a law requiring mandatory retirement, but will make themselves exempt.

- The government has changed the definitions of some of the most basic things we know. Example: There was a reported list of the healthiest states in America. Health, in this particular survey, was defined as the number of hospital beds per 1,000 people, and the percentage of children who got all their recommended vaccinations. They were defining healthiest states as the states where the most people were getting the most amounts of drugs and surgery. How insane. The definition for "spices" now includes thousands of deadly chemicals. Roast beef doesn't have to be real roast beef anymore, it can be a man-made manufactured product and still be called "roast beef."

- Did you know that if you have a child who has been diagnosed with cancer, not giving that child chemotherapy and other drugs can be a criminal offense?

- Politicians who are on the payroll spend 80 percent of their time running for re-election. This is a scam. If a person had a job and decided to run for office, he would not be allowed to take 80 percent of his time and spend it running for office. He would have to resign from his job so he could spend his time in his new pursuit. Politicians, however, stay on the payroll whether they do their job or run for re-election. It's another example of the government out of control.

- The government promotes watchdog groups, but no one is asking who formed these watchdog groups, who started them, who funded them, where do they get their money, what are the salary and perks of its officers and directors. Did you know that most watchdog groups, which appear to be consumer advocate groups or government backed groups, are actually funded by big business, whose objective is to promote the industries or companies that are funding them? These are not watchdog groups at all. They are propaganda organizations used by big business and allowed to flourish by the government.

6. Still not convinced that the FDA is working with big business and major drug companies allowing them to deceive the public and flood the public marketplace with dangerous products? Then consider this:

- Cigarettes are obviously bad; however, they are the only product in America where the ingredients do not have to be listed. How can this be? Well, consider that the FDA is in charge and that the politicians who receive huge amounts of donations and lobbying by the tobacco industry tell the FDA what to do. The obvious connection between the FDA and big tobacco is exposed on the website www.crazyworld.com.

- Federal law prohibits the FDA from using experts with financial conflicts of interest, but the FDA has waived the restriction more than 800 times since 1998. Although the FDA does not reveal when financial conflicts exist, since 1992 it has kept the details of any conflict secret so it is not possible to determine the amount of money or the drug company involved. Two recent articles, both ran in Reuters News and *USA Today,* reported that 54 percent of the experts the FDA asked for advice on which medicines should be approved for sale have a direct financial interest in the drugs or topics they are evaluating. These financial conflicts of interests typically include stock ownership, consulting fees, or research grants. The *USA Today* article stated, "These pharmaceutical experts, about 300 on eighteen different advisory committees, make decisions that affect the health of millions of Americans and billions of billions of dollars in drug sales. With few exceptions, the FDA follows the committee's advice." The scary part is these people who are making these decisions have a direct financial interest and financially benefit based on the decisions they make. The *USA Today* article concluded that at 92 percent of the meetings, at least one member had a financial conflict of interest. At 55 percent of the meetings, half or more of the FDA advisors had conflicts of interest. Conflicts were most frequent at the fifty-seven meetings when broader issues were discussed; 92 percent of those members had conflicts. At the 102 meetings dealing with the fate of a specific drug, 33 percent of the experts had a direct financial interest.

- The pharmaceutical industry has more influence with the FDA than anyone realizes. In the May 19th edition of the prestigious medical journal *Lancet,* editor Richard Horton claimed that the FDA has become a servant to the drug industry. An example: Even though there are multiple deaths caused by certain drugs, the FDA does not recall them from the market, but suggests adding a warning. The LA *Times* reported that the FDA has withheld safety information from labels that physicians say would call into question the use of the drugs. Since 1993, at least 1,000 people were killed by drugs that were approved, but never should have been. Before 1990, 60 percent of drugs submitted to the FDA were approved. Today over 80 percent are approved. *The Los Angeles Times* reported that seven killer drugs that were approved by the FDA, and were so deadly that they had to be withdrawn, generated over $5 billion for the pharmaceutical industry before the recall. Most shocking is that the FDA knowingly puts children at risk. According to the LA *Times* article, the Agency never warned doctors not to administer a drug to infants or other children, even though eight youngsters who were given this drug in clinical studies died. Pediatricians prescribed it widely for infants afflicted with gastric reflux, a common digestive disorder. Patients and their doctors had no way of knowing that the FDA, in August 1996, had found the drug to be "not approvable for children." "We never knew that," said the father of a three-month old son who died on October 28, 1997, after taking the drug. "To me, that means they took my kid as a guinea pig to see if it would work." By the time the drug was pulled, the FDA had received reports of twenty-four deaths of children under age six who had been given this drug. By then, the drug had generated U.S. sales of over $2.5 billion for the drug company.

- An FDA insider said, "People are aware that turning down a drug for approval is going to cause problems with officials higher up in the FDA. Before I came to the FDA, I always assumed things were done properly. I've now lost faith in taking any prescription medication."

- According to the *Los Angeles Times,* "The seven drugs were not needed to save lives. One was for heartburn, another was a diet pill, and a third was a pain killer. All tolled, six of the medicines were never proved to offer life-saving benefits, and the seventh, an antibiotic, was ultimately judged unnecessary because other safer antibiotics were available." These seven drugs have now been found to be so deadly, and have killed so many people, they have all been pulled from the market. The FDA is allowing dangerous drugs to be approved.

- According to the *Los Angeles Times,* in 1988, only 4 percent of new drugs introduced into the world market were approved first by the FDA. In 1998, the FDA's first in the world approval spiked to 66 percent. The reason is now it appears that the easiest agency in the world to approve a new drug, regardless of the safety, is in fact the FDA. The FDA was once the world's leading organization when it came down to the safety of drugs it approved. Now the FDA seems to be more interested in the sales and profits of the drug companies than the safety of consumers. The FDA, as an example, was the last worldwide regulatory agency to withdraw several new drugs in the late 1990s that were banned by health authorities in Europe as being dangerous. Routinely, FDA officials recommend against the approval of drugs, and advisory committees concur and also recommend against the approval of drugs, only to have the drug approved by the FDA and called "safe and effective."

- According to Dr. Kurt D. Furberg, a professor at Wake Forest University, "The patients are the ones paying the price. They're the ones developing all the side effects, fatal and nonfatal."

- One particular drug the FDA approved and called "safe and effective" was pulled within the first year because it was linked to five deaths, the removal of many of the patients' colons, and other major bowel surgeries. Other drugs called "safe and effective" by the FDA had been proven to cause heart valve damage, liver damage, pancreas damage, prostrate cancer, colon cancer, impotency, infertility, heart attack, stroke.

- In the *Los Angeles Times* article, seven specific drugs that were called "safe and effective" resulted in a minimum of 1,000 reported deaths. Other experts say that number is much higher, and could go as high as 20,000 deaths. All from drugs the FDA has called "safe and effective." What is not recorded is the potential hundreds of thousands of patients who took these drugs that developed other severe medical conditions such as liver damage, heart problems, cancer, diabetes, digestive issues, etc. The most outrageous thing is that all of these new medical conditions will be treated by the medical doctors by surgeries and/or more drugs. The needless pain and suffering of hundreds of thousands of people, and the deaths of countless more, is being ignored—all in the name of profit.

- In the *Los Angeles Times* article, it is reported that more than twenty-two million Americans took the drugs that were proven to be dangerous and proven to cause major medical problems. This means there are potentially twenty-two million people who will now have other medical concerns that were caused specifically, and directly, by the drugs they took.

- Dr. Lamuel Loy, a University of Texas School of Public Health physician who served from 1995 to 1999 on the FDA Advisory Committee, says the FDA has lost their compass and forgotten who it is they are ultimately serving.

- The FDA states "All drugs have risks." Most of them have serious risks.

- *The Los Angeles Times* of Tuesday, April 6, 2004, quotes Harvard psychiatrist Dr. Joseph Glen Mullen as saying the following: "Evidence that the FDA is suppressing a report linking suicide to drugs is an outrage given the public health and safety issues at stake." The FDA has information that antidepressants caused children to be twice as likely to show suicidal behavior. The article shows how the FDA claims that there is no conclusive scientific evidence linking antidepressants and potential suicide behavior. However, the article goes on to say that there is absolute evidence that the FDA is suppressing and hiding the information so that the drug companies can continue to sell drugs.

- Nonfatal skin cancers are the number one cancer. The four other most common kinds are breast, prostrate, lung, and colectoral, which is cancer of the colon.

7. Still not convinced that the pharmaceutical industry pushes drug sales and usage at all costs, and has an incestuous desire for increasing profits? Then consider this:

- Nurses are given gifts and money in an attempt to induce them to administer drugs from a specific manufacturer.

- Schools get $500 per month for every child they have on a psychiatric drug, including Ritalin or Prozac.

8. Still not convinced that the ads that you see on television, or read in magazines and newspapers, or hear on the radio are filled with deceptions, fraudulent information, misleading data, and outright lies? Then consider this:

- Ads say things such as "world's finest coffee," "world's best coffee," "best coffee on the planet." These are obviously unsubstantiated and false, but are allowed to run because it's big business.

- TV ads for chain restaurants and fast food restaurants make fraudulent false statements such as "the finest and freshest ingredients" when in fact they are not the finest and freshest ingredients available.

- In restaurants and on television food is shown giving you the impression that when you buy the product it will look like what you see. For anyone who has ever purchased anything, it absolutely never looked like that when it was shown on television, or as it appeared on the package or appeared in the restaurant menu. This is false and misleading, but is allowed to happen because of the lobbyists paying off our friendly politicians.

9. Still not convinced that all over-the-counter nonprescription and prescription drugs are poisons and causing you great physical and emotional harm? Then consider this:

- Depending on who you listen to, either the third or fourth leading cause of death in America is doctors.
- *The Journal of the American Medical Association,* Vol. 284 states, "Things like unnecessary surgery, medical errors, negative effects on drugs, etc., cause almost as many deaths as heart disease and cancer. Over 250,000 people in America alone die each year from physicians' activity or therapy. These account only for the deaths; they do not include people who are permanently maimed, injured, or develop serious other medical conditions due to drugs and surgical procedures. The number of people who get permanent serious disabilities or discomfort, or develop other diseases from drugs and surgical procedures could exceed over three million people per year in America alone."
- Estrogen therapy is now shown to be very dangerous.
- Lowering cholesterol will not prevent a heart attack.
- An aspirin a day can give you a stroke. New research also shows it can destroy your eyesight.
- Sunscreens don't prevent skin cancer, they cause it. Scientists say five ingredients in most sunscreens are highly carcinogenic.
- Since the invention of sunscreen, skin cancer rates in the U.S. have gone up. No one can explain this. No one can explain why

the incidents of skin cancer in the tropical countries where the sun rays are the strongest are very low.

- It has been reported that over seven million Americans older than sixty-five receive prescriptions for drugs that a panel of experts deemed inappropriate for use by the elderly because of potentially dangerous side effects.

- According to a study in the *Journal of the American Medical Association,* every prescription drug has dangerous side effects, and over 20 percent of them come on the market without any warnings.

- In Ralph Nader's book *The Chemical Feast,* he talks about how the Food and Drug Administration deceived consumers and concealed important information about the safety of drugs and food additives. That was over thirty years ago. Amazingly, nothing has changed.

10. Still not convinced that advertising is having a major affect on what you believe and think? Then consider this:

- Advertising has such a profound impact at brainwashing people into believing that drugs and vaccines are so important for health, that if a person does not give their children drugs and vaccines people believe that the children are being neglected and Social Services can take the children away.

- People who have never taken any drugs at all are now going into their doctor and demanding certain drugs that they've seen advertised on television.

- An eighteen year old gets more impressions from drug ads than any other advertising. Over 50,000 drug ads will be exposed to the average eighteen year old.

11. Still not convinced that horror stories in relation to the FDA and the pharmaceutical industry don't exist? Then consider this:

- Alexander Horwin was diagnosed with an aggressive form of brain cancer and underwent two surgeries. The first left him unable to walk, and with optic nerve damage. The second left him tumor free, but his doctors informed him that the disease threatened to return if he didn't receive treatment. The doctors recommended state-of-the-art chemotherapy treatment. It was the best in the world, but the risk included damage to the young infant's heart, lungs, liver and kidneys; and could lead to loss of hearing, small stature, infertility, more cancers, intellectual decline, or even death.

Less than four months after beginning treatment, Alexander died; most probably from the chemotherapy itself. Only later did the parents learn, by reading various medical journals, that the state-of-the-art chemotherapy recommended by the doctors was proven to be ineffective for young children. Various medical journals reported that the drug Alexander was given caused seizures, dementia and death, and even caused cancer itself. This state-of-the-art chemotherapy was performed at a prestigious children's hospital.

The parents found that there were other treatments that were potentially far less dangerous but, according to FDA rules, could not be administered. The parents also found stories of how people with the same disease as their son who received these additional treatments were healthy and suffered few, if any, side effects. The problem was, unbeknownst to the parents, the treatment their son received was part of an FDA approved clinical trial. The FDA regulation that prevented the young infant from receiving the alternative treatment is part of the Food, Drug, and Cosmetics Act, and has been upheld by various lawsuits and state codes. What this means is that Americans don't have the freedom to choose what they and their physicians believe is best. An investigative journalist stated, "Few American are aware that their treatment options, indeed their most personal medical choices, are regulated by the government and are seriously limited if they become ill." This young boy lived only five months after being diagnosed with cancer, yet his medical bills totaled almost $250,000.

- The sad story of Jack and Maryanne Kunari: Their son was diagnosed with brain cancer. Doctors recommended surgery, radiation and chemotherapy, and told the parents of the devastating side effects. The doctors claimed that young Dustin had only four months to live. The parents found an alternative health doctor, Burzynski. When the parents told their medical doctors they were thinking about alternative treatment as an option, they were warned that there was a good chance that social workers from the state could come in and force the young boy to receive the "conventional" treatments of chemotherapy, radiation, surgery and drugs. "It's unbelievable that people have to live with the stress of not only having a severe medical condition in their family, but being threatened that the state will come in, take your son or daughter away from you, and force them to receive horrible, painful medical treatments that will kill them."

- The FDA says patients must use approved therapies, and get no success from those therapies before going to any alternatives. That means that if a person has deadly cancer they must take the poisonous drugs, the radiation and chemotherapy, and pay hundreds of thousands of dollars to the cancer industry, even though these treatments are deadly and could potentially kill them. Luckily for young Dustin, the scenario happened before these laws went into effect, and the parents were not bound by them. The young boy received the alternative all-natural cancer treatments for four years. Eight years later, young Dustin is tumor free, healthy and off medication. You would never know he was sick, his mother said. If this young boy had taken the conventional treatment recommended by the medical doctors of drugs, surgery, radiation, and chemotherapy, the boy would have experienced an excruciatingly painful, horrible existence and probably would have died within a few months anyway.

12. Still not convinced that aspartame (NutraSweet®) is one of the most dangerous food additives available today? Then consider this:

- NutraSweet®, which is aspartame, contains methanol, a wood alcohol which is a deadly poison. Aspartame was approved based on 112 studies submitted to the FDA by the original manufacturer, Surrel Pharmaceuticals, which was acquired by Monsanto. All of these studies were paid for and funded by the drug company. Critics who look at these studies, most notably the fifteen pivotal studies that the FDA based its approval on, are astonished and amazed that anyone could deduce that aspartame is safe. It's amazing that one of the subjects in the study died within a year after taking aspartame. Some of the studies showed people who were taking aspartame were having brain seizures. Once the aspartame was withdrawn from the subjects' diets the brain seizures ceased. All the studies were very short, consisted of only a very few subjects, and the duration was only a few months. The FDA today has received more complaints from people who have consumed aspartame and have had major negative side effects than any other approved food, yet no action has ever been taken.

13. Still not convinced that your thoughts and energy in general is important to your health, and can have a major impact on your physiology, and disease? Then consider this:

   • The magnetic energy of the earth is substantially lower than it has ever been in history. Very few people actually stand with their feet directly on the earth, allowing them to pick up that energy. The earth's gauss, which is measurement of magnetic energy, was at one time 4.0; today it is only .04. The mind and thoughts can have a dramatic instantaneous effect on the body's chemistry and how all organ and gland functions work. In testing people who have been diagnosed with multiple personality disorder, thought has been shown to do what is scientifically impossible. In one particular example, a person's blood was tested and found to be free of diabetes. Within minutes, when his personality changed, the blood was taken again and the person was found to have diabetes. This is physically impossible according to all scientists. It shows that the mind, or the belief system of a person, can do things to the body and change the body chemistry when science has determined that it is impossible to do so. Thoughts and energy absolutely affect a person's physiology and health.

- In research, when a person begins to worry and have stress, the body's pH can go from alkaline to acidic in a matter of minutes. Thoughts can bring on disease faster than any other cause.

- In research, poker players have their body functions monitored, and within a matter of seconds blood pressure and heart rate can dramatically change just by how a person thinks.

- High Definition TVs emit so much powerful electromagnetic energy that in one office building, turning a High Definition TV on wiped out entire computer systems. In addition, High Definition TVs can knock out a bird's natural sense of direction. Electromagnetic waves also have adverse affects on dolphins and whales and their ability to navigate. Certainly then, electromagnetic energy is having a profound negative effect on our physiology and health, as well as our emotional well-being.

- The June 2003 issue of the *Townsend Letter for Doctors and Patients* discussed energy-based frequencies used at clinics throughout the world and how effective they are at curing the incurable diseases.

- According to researchers, electromagnetic frequencies underlie all chemical and mechanical reactions in the body. Applying a frequency that resonates with specific tissues helps the tissue regain coherence and heal. This goes against all medical theories and against the concept that drugs are the only cure and prevention for disease.

- It is actually illegal to use an electromagnetic frequency to heal patients, even though the machine causes absolutely no harm, is nonevasive and painless. However, individual people can own such machines themselves, and use them as they see fit, so long as they do not use the machines to cure a disease. How insane.

- In the owner's manual of a leading computer it says, "Wireless LAN products—like other radio devices—emit radio frequency electromagnetic energy. The level of energy emitted by wireless LAN devices are believed to be safe for use by consumers. These standard recommendations reflect the consensus of the scientific community, and are a result of deliberations of panels and committees of scientists who continually review and interpret the extensive research literature." What this means is that there are many people in the scientific community who believe that wireless based products including radios, computers, global positioning devices, cell phones, etc. emit such powerful and negative electromagnetic energy that it is dangerous for a person to be exposed to these frequencies. Unfortunately, even if you do not own them you are being exposed to these on a regular and consistent basis. It is interesting to note that this so-called warning is put in the owner's manuals of computers.

- Food has energy. The natural energy that natural organic food possesses is vital to the health of the human body. Microwaves dramatically change this energy and make food dangerous to consume. Consider that individual people also emit energy, and can emit energy into food as well. A good example was found at the world famous Rancho Lo Puerta health spa in Mexico. In their organic garden, half of the garden was cultivated and maintained normally. The other half of the garden was also cultivated and maintained normally, but with the addition of having the gardeners consciously emit love to the plants. At the end of the growing season, the half of the garden that was given love produced twice as much crop as the other half. There is no scientific explanation.

- A chiropractor friend of mine had two trees in front of his window. One tree he looked at and emitted love energy. The other tree he looked at and emitted hate and anger energy. In six weeks the tree that received hate and anger energy was withered and almost dead; the other tree was flourishing. Again, there is no scientific explanation.

- My mother and grandmother cooked the exact same Italian pasta with marinara sauce. It looked the same, smelled the same, and was almost identical, but you could always tell who did the cooking. I could never understand how it could taste slightly different. I watched my grandmother cook and I watched my mother cook. They did exactly the same things. They cooked in exactly the same pans in the exact same kitchen. They used the same ingredients and did everything exactly the same way. I could never understand why my mother's cooking tasted different than my grandmother's until I understood that each person emitted a different kind of love energy into the food, which affected the taste of the food.

- While fishing in Canada, our Indian guide would take our freshly caught fish and cook it over an open fire made of wood. The fish was delicious. One day it was raining heavily and we decided to cook inside over gas. The fish was delicious, but tasted different. I asked the Indian guide how that could be. He explained that wood transmitted different energy into the food than the gas flame.

- Energy fields are picked up by all living things on the planet. Whales use energy to navigate the oceans. Salmon are hatched, swim downstream into the ocean, and then have the unbelievable ability to swim back to the exact spot they were hatched to lay their eggs. Birds return to the exact spot after traveling thousands of miles. Science can not explain this because science does not believe in or understand energy fields.

14. Still not convinced that music has a powerful effect on the physiology and your health and wellbeing? Then consider this:

- The latest research confirms that music bypasses your conscious mind. It goes directly to and stimulates the part of the brain that controls your emotions and vital pulses such as heart and respiratory rates, as well as blood pressure. Music that is played at sixty beats or less per minute will slow down your metabolic responses, which not only decreases your stress level, but also increases the amount of chemical endorphins your brain releases and leads to strengthening of your immune system. The exact opposite occurs when listening to music that is against the natural rhythm of the body. Listening to special music that has been designed to work with the body's natural frequency has helped people reduce or eliminate stress, anxiety, pain, insomnia, moodiness, and susceptibility to catching colds and flus, as well as helping to eliminate and prevent many other diseases. It has also been found to turn the body pH from acidic to alkaline, where disease can not exist. Stress reducing music such as this has been proven by healthcare practitioners around the world to be a major aid in eliminating degenerative diseases without drugs and surgery.

15. Still not convinced that research and scientific studies are filled with misrepresentations that are doctored and altered to persuade you to a certain line of thinking, and are in many cases are outright lies and deception? Then consider this:

- According to the FDA's Officer of Inspector General, medical device trials were twice as likely to violate FDA regulations as trials for drugs and biologics. Seventy-five percent of the cited violations included missing data, poor data, and falsification of data. Fraudulent statistics and fraudulent research information is rampant in the healthcare industry.

- Most statistics presented by the medical community are false, misleading and deceptive. Example: In a recent experiment, 100 individuals were sent to psychiatrists for evaluation on whether or not they had attention deficit disorder. These people were incredibly focused, well-balanced, had never been on any psychiatric drugs, incredibly healthy, and maintained high grades in school. The psychiatrist did not know this. They were told simply that they were having some concentration problems and needed a full evaluation. Every single one of these people was diagnosed with attention deficit disorder and prescribed Ritalin or other psychiatric drugs by the psychiatrist. This is fraudulent and outrageous.

- Most studies conducted by the medical industry are specifically designed studies to get the results that the industry wants. Most studies have hand-selected subjects. These subjects are specifically picked out with full knowledge that they will produce the best results. In most studies, the number of subjects can be as small as only five people, and the length of time the study is conducted can be as short as a few weeks. Many pharmaceutical companies do trial studies, figuring out the best way to conduct a study to provide the results they need to get FDA approval of drugs. You simply can not believe any of the studies or research data or alleged "scientific evidence" submitted by the pharmaceutical industry.

16. Still not convinced that the FTC is an unpoliced, unregulated independent government agency that actually is judge, jury, and executioner, suppressing the rights of Americans while protecting the profits of big business? Then consider this:

- There are so many stories of how the FTC has attacked companies selling alternative healthcare remedies that are harmless and absolutely work. One company had a product that reduced or eliminated pain in over 90 percent of the subjects tried. Over 18,000 people had used this product with spectacular results. But because the pain industry is so profitable, this product was squashed by the FTC and virtually banned from the market.

- The government spends tens of millions of dollars prosecuting people and small companies who do not have the resources to defend themselves. It's David versus Goliath. If you are sued by the government, you don't have a chance.

- The FTC admits that it usually does not, and the FDA does not, receive any reports of people injured by products being sold that they attack and go after.

- David Walker was found to have cancer, and was told by his doctor he had no more than three to five years before his colon cancer would kill him. Twelve years later, Walker is cancer free. Walker cured himself. He created his own treatment, which includes herbs, enzymes, vital nutrients, detoxification and energetic therapy that recharged the depleted cells, alkalized his body and allowed his cancer to vanish. He shared his knowledge and helped hundreds of other cancer patients eliminate their disease without drugs or surgery. But the Federal Trade Commission sued Mr. Walker, citing as its basis Walker's records reporting that 14 percent of the people using his protocol died. However, the report did not include the mortality rate over the same period for cancer patients who underwent the approved cancer therapies—drugs, radiation and chemotherapy. In that group **96 percent** of the people using that protocol died. When the court case ended, Walker became one of the thousands of individuals and companies whose effective alternative nondrug and nonsurgical health treatments have been stifled. You can read the entire story on www.sumeria.net.

  The article claims that an individual with breast cancer used Walker's regime and her cancer was cured. When she informed her physician, the doctor claimed to have lost $350,000 because her breast cancer went away. The Federal Trade Commission, under pressure from the FDA, then went to work. Never mind that Walker had over 2,500 testimonials from people who loved his protocol. Eighty-six percent of the people that Walker worked with survived their cancers. The government did not care. The only thing that they cared about was that he was not using approved drugs, surgery, and radiation.

17. Still not convinced that organic food is much better for you? Then consider this:

    - A February 2003 study published in the *Journal of Agriculture and Food Industry* showed organically grown berries contain up to 58 percent more polyphenolics than those grown conventionally. This means that organically grown berries have 58 percent more antioxidants than those grown conventionally.

- A 1993 study published in the *Journal of Applied Nutrition,* showed that over the course of two years organic foods contained up to four times as many trace minerals, thirteen times more selenium and twenty times more calcium and magnesium than commercially produced produce, and also had significantly fewer heavy metals, including 25 percent less lead and 40 percent less aluminum.

18. Still not convinced that we are losing the war on cancer and cancer is getting worse and worse every year? Then consider this:

- Nonfatal skin cancers are the number-one form of cancer. The four other most common kinds are breast cancer, prostrate, lung, and cancer of the colon.

- Cancer will surpass heart disease as the number-one cause of death in the United States in the next few years. Every year, over 1.5 million Americans are diagnosed with cancer and the number is increasing. The probability that you will develop cancer is one in every two men and one in every three women, and it's getting worse. The war on cancer has been a total failure. Some scientists estimate that up to 70 percent of all cancers could be prevented simply by dietary change. The only legal remedies for cancer treatment are surgery, chemotherapy, and radiation. You can go to jail if you treat cancer with all-natural methods even though they are more effective than surgery, chemotherapy and radiation, and have absolutely no negative side effects. This is insane.

Still not convinced that the FDA suppresses information on natural cures? Then consider this:

- *The California Western Law Review* published an article entitled "Why Does the FDA Deny Access to Alternative Cancer Treatments?"

- Canadian scientist, Gaston Naessens, created an herbal blend called 714-X. This blend, as of 1991, has cured more than 1,000 people of cancer, as well as several AIDS patients. The FDA has attacked him. The story is on website http://www. luminet.net/~wenonah/new/naessen.htm.

- Jason Winter authored the book *Killing Cancer,* which has sold more than a million copies, about how he cured his cancer with herbs. He is quoted as saying, "I must tell you that I was scared about publishing a book talking about how herbs can cure cancer. I was not prepared to take on the billion dollar drug companies, the medical associations and doctors, all of whom would chew up and spit out anyone that would dare to say that possibly, just possibly, herbs can help." Winters outlines the typical fate of natural cancer and other cures that are advertised in U.S. publications. Usually the publication gets into a lot of trouble for printing it in the first place, and then all future publicity is stopped. The persons selling the products are usually tricked or entrapped into a phony suit about "practicing medicine without a license," or "selling drugs without a license," or selling "unregistered drugs." If the government can't stop them that way, they usually use another federal agency, the IRS, to attack them with some phony, trumped up income tax charge. Those who practice natural medicine, or sell natural remedies, live with the knowledge that they could be closed down any day.

- Registered nurse, Kathy Stevens, promotes the benefits of magnets. However, she is forbidden from using the word "pain." She must only use the word "discomfort," otherwise she is selling an unregistered medical device without a license and making a medical claim that is unsubstantiated. Kathy herself suffered from osteoarthritis pain for five years. Her brother exposed her to a nondrug solution. Being a registered nurse, she was trained only in drugs and surgery. When her brother suggested that she try magnets, she laughed and scoffed. According to the medical establishment, magnets do nothing to reduce or eliminate pain or have any other health benefits. The medical community states that there is no credible scientific evidence showing that magnets have any health benefits whatsoever. While at a family reunion, her brother had her sleep on a magnetic sleeping pad and a pillow, as well as a quilt containing far inferred technology. Kathy recounts waking up the next morning astonished that she had slept the entire night without waking. She experienced absolutely no pain for the first time in five years. She couldn't believe that she was pain free and her body was full of energy. Kathy believes, based on her own personal experience, and that of witnessing countless others, that anyone's osteoarthritis pain can be reduced or eliminated by the use of magnets. She can't tell people the truth, and she can't tell people what she has experienced for herself or witnessed. If she does, she could be prosecuted and potentially arrested and jailed. In effect, she has lost her right of free speech because her opinions go against the monopoly of the pharmaceutical industry.

• Keep in mind that the FDA wants to prosecute anyone who is curing disease without the use of drugs and surgery. The tens of thousands of alternative/natural healthcare practitioners are risking their very existences—not because of riches, but because of genuine concern for people's health and wellbeing. It is sad to know that millions of people suffer needlessly because of the government's suppression of natural alternatives.

• It pains me knowing that people die every year because of the government's suppression of the truth about all-natural alternatives and the dangers of drugs and surgery. These doctors or healthcare practitioners will generally say they do not cure anything. In many cases they say they do not treat cancer and they do not treat any form of disease, because saying so would put them in peril with the FDA. They are acting as an underground organization, doing so because of their mission for the betterment of mankind. Many times when you see an alternative healthcare practitioner they will have you sign a whole host of forms, disclaimers, release forms, and statements asserting that they are not trying to cure or prevent any disease, and that you are seeing them under your own free will. Because of our litigious society, and because of the oppression imposed by the government regulating bodies, these wonderful individuals, by risking so much, must take these measures in order to protect their ability to treat people who need their treatment.

- In a *New York Times* news service article, it was stated that more than half of all new drugs approved for marketing have severe or fatal side effects not found in testing, and not reported until years after the medications have been widely used. This information was found by congressional investigators. The General Accounting Office showed that between 1976 and 1985, of 198 drugs approved, over half of them should be taken off the market because they are so deadly and caused so many medical problems. This again shows that taking any nonprescription or prescription drug absolutely causes medical problems. The drugs themselves give you illness, sickness and disease.

- Virtually all violent acts committed by children in schools over the last ten years were committed by individuals who had been on prescribed psychiatric drugs. The psychiatric drugs prescribed increase the chance of suicide and dramatically increase the chance of violent acts. Prescribed psychiatric drugs are deadly and should never be consumed.

- Most drugs are physically addicting. Most notably, pain medication, as evidenced by many celebrities, including Rush Limbaugh, who were given drugs by their doctor not knowing the addictive nature of the drug. Unable to stop, these people became slaves to the drug. The drugs also caused major medical problems such as permanent hearing loss.

19. Still not convinced that government agencies fight against individuals while allowing big business to go unpoliced? Then consider this:

- The IRS audits three times the percentage of individuals as opposed to corporations, small businesses, and partnerships. The largest multinational corporations get audited the least even though they are the ones most likely of committing tax fraud.

20. Still not convinced that "experts" are generally wrong when they present things as fact when they should be presenting it as opinion, or that these "experts" are paid spokespeople and have a financial interest and conflict of interest in relation to what they are saying? Then consider this:

- Talent agents give their expert opinion as fact as to who has talent and who will never make it. However, most talent agents have been proven to be wrong more often than they are right. Examples: Britney Spears lost in her appearance in Star Search. Elvis Presley was told by a talent scout that he had no talent and should go back to driving a truck. Most major actors, actresses, and musicians were told by experts that they should give up and they had no talent.

- The president of Digital Equipment Corporation said that there was absolutely no long-term market for a home personal computer. He was obviously wrong to such a huge degree that the statement sounds insane. Surprisingly, this person made the statement in the late 1970s.

- The USDA has daily recommended allowances of nutrients. These are taken by the American public as factual and scientifically based. The USDA can not give any scientific basis or rational reason how these numbers have been established. Throughout the last fifty years these daily recommended requirements have changed radically. The point is that just because a government agency says you need this or you don't need something else doesn't mean it's true. Generally speaking, history shows that they are wrong.

- Government agencies tell you the nutrients you need in your diet, and in what levels. However, every few years new nutrients are discovered. Just because a nutrient hasn't been discovered doesn't mean you don't need it. This is one of the major reasons why whole food supplements are so much better than chemical or synthetic vitamins. It is also the reason why studies and research done on synthetic vitamins do not necessarily show favorable results. When studies are conducted with whole food concentrates, whole food concentrates that include not only the vitamin in question, but all the cofactors and parts and elements that defy analysis, the results are always better. Remember, science is not better than nature.

21. Still not convinced that you are under massive amounts of physiological, energetic, and emotional stress that are affecting your health and causing your body to be acidic, which leads to virtually all disease? Then consider this:

- I was fishing in Canada with my good friend Dr. Morter, one of the pioneers in pH research. After our third day of fishing in a stress-free environment with no telephones, no computers, no TVs, virtually in the middle of nowhere, he told me that every person has locked in stress that is adversely affecting their health. I told him I was totally relaxed and didn't think I had any stress. He then said to me, "Relax the muscles in your forehead," which I promptly did. He then pointed out if I was totally relaxed, how could I relax muscles in my forehead? You see, if I was totally relaxed the muscles in my forehead would have actually been relaxed and could not have been relaxed any further. The fact was, I was holding them tight unconsciously. We are all under massive amounts of stress in today's living environment. This stress causes our body pH to become acidic, setting up the perfect environment for sickness and disease. It is vital that you de-stress and relax on a regular basis. De-stressing and relaxing on a regular basis has been shown to reverse virtually every disease because the state of full relaxation puts your body in a state of alkaline pH where disease can not exist.

22. Not convinced that you need to eat more raw, uncooked organic fruits, vegetables, nuts and seeds? Then consider this:

    • Dogs who ate standard man-made, chemically laced produced dog food live, depending on the breed, between twelve and fourteen years. Dogs that are fed all organic raw food, as they would eat in nature, live to be twenty-two to thirty years old.

23. Not convinced that companies produce poisons that they call "food"? Then consider this:

    • People always ask me, "Why do food companies and restaurants put all of these chemicals into the food?" The answer is very simple, they must make the food in the cheapest possible manner. This means growing the food in an unnatural way, which produces food that virtually has no taste. The food can not be allowed to spoil, as it would cost the company money. It is laced with chemicals to make the food last a very long time. In the processing of the food, chemicals are put in to make you physically addicted to the food, to make you hungrier by increasing your appetite, and are specifically design to make you fat. This increases sales and profits for the food companies. Companies also have to produce food that can have a shelf life of many years, so that it can be stored if it is not sold and the company can still make a profit. Real, whole, natural food virtually has no shelf life; it goes rancid, therefore is not profitable to the food companies. Remember my earlier example of how homogenization and pasteurization replaced the milkman.

    The processing of food itself turns the food from real food that nourishes and feeds the body into something that is foreign to the body, unnatural and causes the body undue physiological stress to cope. It causes disease and makes you age faster. For years, the food industry has refused to list the amount of trans fats on the label. A cost benefit analysis conducted in 1999 by the FDA itself showed savings of $8 billion per year in averted heart disease costs alone, and a saving of 5,000 American lives if trans fats were listed on the label. In fact, you could say the FDA's failure to require the food companies to list trans fats caused the death of 5,000 Americans. Maybe the FDA should be listed as a terrorist organization?

Have you noticed how the news has changed? Today, the lead news story is what happened on last night's reality TV series. Doesn't this amaze you? Well, consider that the news organizations own the networks that produce the reality TV shows; it is no wonder that they are more interested in promoting their other businesses, disguising it as news, than adhering to their journalistic responsibilities as news broadcasters. Remember, it's always about the money.

I was told by an insider that a major hamburger chain has to put chemical flavorings in their hamburgers so that they actually taste like hamburgers.

My most recent experience of how healthcare is really a monopoly for the pharmaceutical industry was when I requested some blood tests be done. I walked in to a lab and asked for some blood work to be performed. I was told it was against the law to do blood work without a prescription. I was appalled how the lawmakers created this monopoly for medical doctors. I reluctantly acquired a prescription. When I had my blood drawn I paid the bill and asked when I could get my results. I was told it was against the law for them to give me my test results. It must be sent to a medical doctor. This was my blood, and I paid for the tests with my money, yet the law denies me direct access to the results. This is a good example of how lawmakers guarantee profits for medical doctors.

Some people wonder if corporate executives are as ruthless and greedy as I suggest many of them are. Consider Ford Motor Company. The executives knew that if they did not recall the Ford Pinto hundreds of people would die. Yet they made the decision not to order the recall because it would cost too much money. They decided that profits were more important than people dying or being maimed for life.

Can such corruption actually be occurring in the corporate world, with politicians and government agencies, on such a widespread basis without anyone blowing the whistle? Consider the New York police officer Frank Serpico. A movie and book came out about his life. For years payoffs, bribes, and corruption were widespread and common-place in the New York police department. It went to the highest levels. Yet for years no one exposed the truth and no one even considered that such corruption could be occurring on such a widespread basis for so long within law enforcement. However, when the truth was exposed the unthinkable and unimaginable had been occurring. Right now, this same type of corruption is occurring in healthcare at every level.

C H A P T E R   1 1

Still Not Convinced?

This book contains many basic premises. Some, or probably most, of my statements may be hard to believe. Some of the things I say, such as walking being incredibly healthy, or eating more fresh, raw fruit and vegetables has many health benefits, may be easy to accept. Other basic premises that I espouse in this book, such as nonprescription and prescription drugs cause disease, may be harder to accept as true. I encourage you to educate yourself on these subjects. To help you do that, I would like to provide additional material that goes into detail on these various subjects. Much of this material is authored by, surprisingly enough, medical doctors who were trained in surgery and the prescribing of drugs. They know the truth firsthand from an insider's perspective. Other authors come directly from the industry that they are writing about. All of this material is available by calling 800-931-4721, or going to www.naturalcures.com. If you do purchase any of these books, CDs or videotapes, I do make a small profit. However, if you purchase any other product I recommend, in the spirit of full disclosure, please know that I do **not** receive any compensation. There is no financial incentive for me to recommend any product or service. As far as I know, I am one of the only authors who is not compensated financially on the sale of products he recommends. I do this to let you know my recommendations are what I absolutely believe in my heart to be the best for you. My mission is to be a guiding force in helping people all over the world be healthy. Please buy your books from us to help support this mission.

1. NOT CONVINCED THAT PASTEURIZED AND HOMOGENIZED MILK IS DEADLY? NOT CONVINCED THAT YOU SHOULD ONLY BE EATING ORGANIC, RAW, UNPASTEURIZED AND UNHOMOGENIZED DAIRY PRODUCTS? THEN READ:

   - *Homogenized Milk May Cause Your Heart Attack: The XO Factor*
   (and how it can destroy your arteries, your heart, your life!)

   - *Don't Drink Your Milk!*
   (New frightening medical facts about the world's most overrated nutrient.)

   - *MILK—The Deadly Poison*

2. NOT CONVINCED THAT ASPARTAME (NUTRASWEET®) AND MONOSODIUM GLUTAMATE (MSG) ARE DEADLY AND SHOULD NEVER BE CONSUMED? THEN READ:

   - *ASPARTAME (NutraSweet®) Is It Safe?*

   - *EXCITOTOXINS—The Taste that Kills*
   (How monosodium glutamate, aspartame [NutraSweet®] and similar substances can cause harm to the brain and nervous system, and their relationship to neurodegenerative diseases such as Alzheimer's, Lou Gehrig's disease (ALS) and others.)

   - *IN BAD TASTE: The MSG Symptom Complex*

3. NOT CONVINCED THAT YOU HAVE A CANDIDA YEAST OVERGROWTH CAUSING ALL TYPES OF MEDICAL PROBLEMS INCLUDING EXCESS WEIGHT, ARTHRITIS, DEPRESSION, PMS, ACNE, MIGRAINES, STRESS, CONSTIPATION, BLOATING, SKIN RASHES AND MORE? THEN READ:

   - *Lifeforce*
   (A dynamic plan for health, vitality and weight loss.)

4. NOT CONVINCED THAT SUBTLE ENERGY THERAPIES CAN CURE VIRTUALLY ALL DISEASE? THEN READ:

   - *Sanctuary*
   (The Path to Consciousness)

- *Vibrational Medicine*
  (The #1 handbook of subtle energy therapies.)
- *Energy Medicine—The Scientific Basis*

5. NOT CONVINCED THAT FOOD ADDITIVES ARE A LEADING CAUSE OF ILLNESS? THEN READ:

- *Hard to Swallow*
  (The Truth About Food Additives.)

6. NOT CONVINCED THE FOOD INDUSTRY IS PURPOSELY CREATING FOODS THAT MAKE YOU PHYSICALLY ADDICTED, INCREASE YOUR APPETITE, MAKE YOU FAT AND GIVE YOU DISEASE? THEN READ:

- *Fast Food NATION—The Dark Side of the All-American Meal*
- *The Crazy Makers*
  (How the Food Industry Is Destroying Our Brains and Harming our Children.)
- *Genetically Engineered Food—Changing the Nature of Nature*
  (What You Need to Know to Protect Yourself, Your Family, and Our Planet)
- *Food Politics*
  (How the Food Industry Influences Nutrition and Health.)
- *Restaurant CONFIDENTIAL*
  (Think a chicken Caesar salad is perfect for your diet? Think again. Choose a tuna sandwich over the roast beef sandwich? Wrong! The startling truth about our favorite foods from our favorite restaurants, with fat, calorie and salt content.)
- *FAT LAND*
  (How Americans Became the Fattest People in the World.)

7. NOT CONVINCED THAT VACCINES ARE DEADLY, CAUSE DISEASE AND SHOULD NEVER BE USED? THEN READ:

- *A Shot in the Dark*
  (Why the P in the DPT vaccination may be hazardous to your child's health.)

- *VACCINES: Are They Really Safe & Effective?*
- *What Your Doctor May Not Tell You About Children's Vaccinations*

8. NOT CONVINCED THAT CANCER CAN BE CURED WITHOUT DRUGS AND SURGERY? THEN READ:
   - *The Cancer Cure That Worked! Fifty Years of Suppression*
   - *The Cancer Conspiracy*
   - *How to Fight Cancer & Win*
     (Scientific guidelines and documented facts for the successful treatment and prevention of cancer and other related health problems.)
   - *The Breuss Cancer Cure*
     (Advice for the prevention and natural treatment of cancer, leukemia and other seemingly incurable diseases.)
   - *The Cancer Industry*
     (The Classic Exposé on the Cancer Establishment.)
   - *The Cure for All Cancers*
     (New research findings show there is a single cause for all cancers. This book provides exact instructions for their cure.)
   - *The Healing of Cancer—The Cures—the Cover-ups and the Solution Now*

9. NOT CONVINCED THAT STRESS CAUSES YOUR BODY TO BECOME ACIDIC AND, WHEN HANDLED, THAT VIRTUALLY ALL DISEASES CAN BE CURED? THEN READ:
   - *Stress: The Silent Killer*

10. NOT CONVINCED THAT YOUR THOUGHTS CAN MAKE YOU SICK OR HEAL YOU? THEN READ:
    - *Anatomy of an Illness as Perceived by the Patient*
      (Reflections on Healing and Regeneration.)
    - *Why Animals Don't Get Heart Attacks...But People Do!*
      The Discovery that will Eradicate Heart Disease
      (The natural prevention of heart attacks, strokes, high blood

pressure, diabetes, high cholesterol, and many other cardiovascular conditions.)

- *HEAD FIRST—The Biology of Hope and Healing Power of the Human Spirit*

11. NOT CONVINCED THAT YOU SHOULD NEVER EAT ANY MEAT OR POULTRY THAT IS NOT ORGANIC? THEN READ:

- *Slaughterhouse*
  (The Shocking Story of Greed, Neglect, and Inhumane Treatment Inside the U.S. Meat Industry.)

- *Mad Cow*
  (Plain Truth from the Cattle Rancher Who Won't Eat Meat.)

- *Prisoned Chickens, Poisoned Eggs*
  (An Inside Look at the Modern Poultry Business.)

12. NOT CONVINCED THAT OUR FOOD IS LOADED WITH CHEMICALS CAUSING ILLNESS AND DISEASE? THEN READ:

- *The Chemical Feast*
  (Ralph Nader's Study Group Report on the Food and Drug Administration.)

- *A Chemical Feast*
  (A rational, commonsense discussion of chemicals in foods by a noted specialist in nutrition and epidemiology.)

- *Sowing the Wind*
  (A report from Ralph Nader's Center for Study of Responsive Law on Food Safety and the Chemical Harvest.)

13. NOT CONVINCED THAT ELECTROMAGNETIC POLLUTION IS BOMBARDING YOUR BODY, CAUSING ALL KINDS OF MEDICAL PROBLEMS? THEN READ:

- *Cross Currents—*
  The Promise of Electromedicine

- *Electromagnetic Fields*
  (A Consumer's Guide to the Issues and How to Protect Ourselves.)

14. NOT CONVINCED THAT WE ALL HAVE AN ENERGETIC FIELD AROUND US THAT IS ADVERSELY AFFECTED BY MAGNETIC POLLUTION? THEN READ:

- *The Unseen Self*

   (Kirlian Photography Explained.)

- *Kirlian Photography—A Hands-On Guide*

15. NOT CONVINCED THAT DRUGS ARE POISONS AND CAUSE MOST DISEASE? THEN READ:

- *Over Dose*
   The Case Against the Drug Companies—Prescription Drugs, Side Effects, and Your Health

- *Bitter Pills*
   Inside the Hazardous World of Legal Drugs

16. NOT CONVINCED THAT THE PHARMACEUTICAL INDUSTRY IS PURPOSELY SELLING INEFFECTIVE DANGEROUS DRUGS, AND WORKING TIRELESSLY TO SUPPRESS NATURAL, EFFECTIVE CURES FOR DISEASE? THEN READ:

- *Racketeering in Medicine—The Suppression of Alternatives*

- *The Drug Lords*
   America's Pharmaceutical Cartel

- *The Big Fix*
   (How the Pharmaceutical Industry Rips Off American Consumers)

- *The Assault on Medical Freedom*
   (Why American Healthcare are Costs So Much!)

- *Disease-Mongers—How Doctors, Drug Companies, and Insurers Are Making You Feel Sick*

- *Under the Influence of Modern Medicine*

- *The Social Transformation of American Medicine*
   (The rise of a sovereign profession and the making of a vast industry.)

- *Confessions of a Medical Heretic*
   (Approximately 2.4 million operations performed every year are unnecessary and cost about 12,000 lives. In six New York

hospitals, 43 percent of performed hysterectomies reviewed were found to be unjustified. Historically, when doctors have gone on strike, the mortality rate has dropped.)

- *Medical Blunders*
  (Amazing True Stories of Mad, Bad, and Dangerous Doctors.)

17. NOT CONVINCED THAT PSYCHIATRY, PSYCHOLOGY, AND ALL PSYCHIATRIC DRUGS HARM PATIENTS AND ACTUALLY CAUSE DEPRESSION, SUICIDE, VIOLENT ACTS, AND DISEASE? THEN READ:

- *Psychiatry: The Ultimate Betrayal*

- *Your Drug May Be Your Problem*
  (How and Why to Stop Taking Psychiatric Medications.)

- *Talking Back To Ritalin*
  (What Doctors Aren't Telling You About Stimulants and ADHD.)

- *Talking Back To Prozac*
  (What doctors aren't telling you about today's most controversial drug.—The only book that tells you the truth behind its testing and it's potentially frightening side effects.)

- *The Antidepressant Fact Book*
  (What Your Doctor Won't Tell You About Prozac, Zoloft, Paxil, Celexa, and Luvox.)

- *The Myth of Mental Illness*
  (Foundations of a Theory of Personal Conduct.)

- *The Manufacture of Madness*
  (A Comparative Study of the Inquisition and the Mental Health Movement.)

- *Mad in America*
  (Bad Science, Bad Medicine, and the Enduring Mistreatment of the Mentally Ill.)

18. NOT CONVINCED THAT CALCIUM IS A NUTRIENT THAT MOST PEOPLE ARE DEPLETED IN? THEN READ:

- *The Calcium Factor: The Scientific Secret of Health and Youth.*
  (The Relationship Between Nutrient Deficiency And Disease.)

19. NOT CONVINCED THAT IF YOUR BODY pH IS ALKALINE YOU CAN VIRTUALLY NEVER GET SICK? THEN READ:

- *Alkalize or Die*
  (Superior Health Through Proper Alkaline-Acid Balance.)
- *Dynamic Health*
  (Using Your Own Beliefs, Thoughts And Memory To Create A Healthy Body.)
- *The Acid-Alkaline Diet for Optimum Health*
  (Restore Your Health By Creating Balance In Your Diet.)
- *The pH Miracle*
  (Balance Your Diet, Reclaim Your Health.)

20. NOT CONVINCED THAT MAGNETS CAN HEAL, ALLEVIATE PAIN, AND CURE DISEASE? THEN READ:

- *Magnet Therapy*
  (The Gentle and Effective Way to Balance Body Systems.)
- *Healing with Magnets*
  ("Study on Using Magnets to Treat Pain Surprises Skeptics" — *New York Times)*

21. NOT CONVINCED THAT AIDS IS ONE OF THE GREATEST HOAXES AND DECEPTIONS EVER PERPETRATED ON THE AMERICAN PUBLIC? THEN READ:

- *AIDS*
  (The good news is HIV doesn't cause it. The bad news is "recreational drugs" and medical treatments like AZT do.)
- *Inventing the AIDS Virus*
- *AIDS: What the Government Isn't Telling You*
- *Infectious AIDS: Have We Been Misled?*
  (A collection of thirteen articles originally published in scientific journals that call into question the dogma of infectious AIDS.)
- *The AIDS War*
  (Propaganda, Profiteering and Genocide from the Medical-Industrial Complex.)

- *Do Insects Transmit AIDS?*

- *Why We Will Never Win the War on AIDS*
  (Greed, power, sex, and politics have combined to create the biggest SCAM in medical history: AIDS. But now, everything you thought you knew about this "deadly epidemic" is about to change...)

22. NOT CONVINCED THAT YOUR DIGESTIVE SYSTEM IS ABSOLUTELY DYSFUNCTIONAL IF YOU LIVE IN AMERICA? THEN READ:

- *Restoring Your Digestive Health*
  (How the Guts and Glory Program Can Transform Your Life.)

23. NOT CONVINCED THAT STRESS, ANXIETY, AND EMOTIONAL PROBLEMS CAN BE CURED ALMOST INSTANTLY? THEN READ:

- *7 Steps to Overcoming Depression and Anxiety*
  (A practical Guide to Mental, Physical, and Spiritual Wellness.)

- *The Basic DIANETICS Picture Book*
  (A visual aid to a better understanding of man and the mind based on the works of L. Ron Hubbard.)

- *Scientology Picture Book*
  (Use it to understand yourself, life, and those you live with.)

- *Dianetics*
  (The Modern Science of Mental Health.)

24. NOT CONVINCED THAT PAIN IN ANY PART OF YOUR BODY CAN BE ELIMINATED EASILY WITHOUT DRUGS OR SURGERY? THEN READ:

- *Pain Free: An Evolutionary Method for Stopping Chronic Pain*

- *Instant Relief: Tell Me Where it Hurts and I'll Tell You What to Do*

- *Pain Free at Your PC*
  (Using a computer doesn't have to hurt. Prevent or reverse repetitive stress injuries; cure carpal tunnel syndrome; end chronic wrist, shoulder, and neck pain; ease eyestrain; avoid surgery, drugs, and wrist braces.)

- *Natural Relief from Aches & Pains*
  (Alternatives to Over-the-Counter Medications for many conditions.)

25. NOT CONVINCED THAT WOMEN ARE BEING EXPLOITED BY THE MEDICAL ESTABLISHMENT? THEN READ:

- *The Politics of Stupid*
  (Lose the weight you want to lose forever.)

- *Hormone Replacement Therapy: Yes or No?*
  (How To Make An Informed Decision About Estrogen, Progesterone & Other Strategies For Dealing With PMS, Menopause, And Osteoporosis.

- *Alternative Medicine Guide to Women's Health*
  (Clinically Proven Alternative Therapies for Relief From Women's Health Conditions . . .)

- *Male Practice: How Doctors Manipulate Women*

26. NOT CONVINCED THAT TAP WATER CONTAINING FLUORIDE, CHLORINE AND OTHER CONTAMINANTS IS A MAJOR CAUSE OF ILLNESS AND DISEASE? THEN READ:

- *Fluoride: The Aging Factor*
  (How to Recognize and Avoid the Devastating Effects of Fluoride. Find Out Who's Profiting from the Chronic Poisoning of Over 130 million Americans!)

- *Your Body's Many Cries For Water*
  (You are not sick, you are thirsty! Don't treat thirst with medications—A preventative and self-education manual for those who prefer to adhere to the logic of the natural and the simple in medicine.)

- *Don't Drink The Water*
  (The Essential Guide to Our Contaminated Drinking Water and What You Can Do About It.)

- *Water—The Foundation of Youth, Health, and Beauty*

- *The Water We Drink*
  (Water Quality And Its Effects On Health.)

- *The Drinking Water Book*
  (A Complete Guide to Safe Drinking Water. There's nothing more important than the quality of the water that you drink.)

- *Water: for Health, for Healing, for Life*
  (You're not sick, you're thirsty! You always knew water was good for you. Now discover why it's nature's miracle

- *Water Wasteland*
  (Ralph Nader's Study Group Report on Water Pollution.)

27. NOT CONVINCED THAT ARTHRITIS CAN BE ELIMINATED WITHOUT ANY DRUGS OR SURGERY? THEN READ:

- *Arthritis Defeated at Last! The Real Arthritis Cure*
  (The amazing story of CMO™—Nature's revolutionary immuno-modulator that rectifies the cause of arthritis forever!)

- *Arthritis Beaten Today!*
  (A revolutionary, new, natural, dietary supplement that is restoring the quality of life of people suffering from arthritis, as well as other chronic autoimmune diseases. The CMO™ story is a scientific breakthrough that has been described as "The nutritional discovery of the 20th century.")

28. NOT CONVINCED THAT REBOUNDING EXERCISES STRENGTH-EN EVERY CELL IN THE BODY, AND BRING VIBRANT HEALTH AND WEIGHT LOSS? THEN READ:

- *Looking Good, Feeling Great*
  (Fifteen Minutes a Day to a New You. An easy, fun way to tone you figure, improve health, and develop total fitness!)

- *Rebounding to Better Health*
  (A Practical Guide to the Ultimate Exercise.)

- *Urban Rebounding™. . . An Exercise for The New Millennium*
  (The system known as Urban Rebounding brings together the science of the West and the philosophy and practicality of the East to form a holistic program of exercise in which people of all ages, sizes, shapes and states of physical condition can participate.)

- *Harry and Sarah Sneider's Olympic Trainer*
  (The world's finest total body fitness system that's easy and fun for everyone! Improves: gripping, throwing, jumping, kicking, sprinting, skiing, skating, stamina, depth perception, balance, coordination, body alignment and endurance.)

29. NOT CONVINCED THAT THE FDA IS PURPOSELY SUPPRESSING NATURAL CURES FOR DISEASES, AND ALLOWS DRUG MANU-FACTURERS TO SELL INEFFECTIVE AND DANGEROUS DRUGS? THEN READ:

    - *Innocent Casualties: The FDA's War Against Humanity*

    - *Stop the FDA: Save Your Health Freedom*
      (Discover the FDA's hidden agenda; learn how to improve your health with supplements; discover the real reasons the FDA banned tryptophan; find out how the FDA suppresses medical breakthroughs; learn the true value of nutritional medicine; learn what you can do to save you health freedom.)

    - *Hazardous to Our Health?*
      (FDA Regulation of Healthcare Products.)

    - *Protecting America's Health*
      (The FDA, Business, and One Hundred Years of Regulation.)

    - *The History of a Crime Against the Food Law*
      (The Amazing Story Of The National Food And Drugs Law Intended To Protect The Health Of The People—Perverted To Protect Adulteration of Foods And Drugs.)

30. NOT CONVINCED THAT USING OXYGEN CAN REVERSE AGING, SPEED HEALING, AND POTENTIALLY CURE MANY DISEASES? THEN READ:

    - *Flood Your Body with Oxygen*
      (Therapy for our polluted world.)

    - *Stop Aging or Slow the Process: Exercise With Oxygen Therapy (EWOT) Can Help*

    - *Oxygen Healing Therapies*
      (For Optimum Health & Vitality, Bio-Oxidative Therapies for

Treating Immune Disorders, Candida, Cancer, Heart, Skin, Circulatory & Other Modern Diseases.)

31. NOT CONVINCED THAT YOGA HAS ABSOLUTELY AMAZING HEALTH BENEFITS? THEN READ:

- *Ancient Secret of The Fountain of Youth*
  (Can five ancient Tibetan rites really make you look and feel years younger? The secret of youthful health and vitality.)

- *Bikram's Beginning Yoga Class*
  (Classic Illustrated Yoga Guide.)

- *Power Yoga*
  (The Total Strength and Flexibility Workout.)

32. NOT CONVINCED THAT YOU CAN ELIMINATE PHOBIAS, TRAU-MAS, ADDICTIONS AND COMPULSIONS IN AS LITTLE AS FIVE MINUTES? THEN READ:

- *Tapping the Healer Within*
  (Using Thought Field Therapy to Instantly Conquer Your Fears, Anxieties, and Emotional Distress.)

33. NOT CONVINCED THAT HERBAL REMEDIES CAN POTENTIAL-LY CURE MANY DISEASES? THEN READ:

- *Next Generation Herbal Medicine*
  (Guaranteed Potency Herbs.)

- *Herbal Tonic Therapies*
  (Remedies from nature's own pharmacy to strengthen and support each vital body system.)

- *Herbal Healing: An Easy to Use A-Z Reference*

34. NOT CONVINCED THAT HOMEOPATHIC MEDICINES ARE A SAFE NATURAL ALTERNATIVE TO DRUGS AND SURGERY AND CAN CURE DISEASE AND KEEP YOU HEALTHY? THEN READ:

- *Everybody's Guide to Homeopathic Medicines*
  (Safe And Effective Remedies For You And Your Family. Homeopathy is a natural, safe, inexpensive, and highly effective complement to conventional medicine.)

- *The Complete Homeopathy Handbook*
  (Safe and effective ways to treat fevers, coughs, colds and sore throats, childhood ailments, food poisoning, flu, and a wide range of everyday complaints.)

35. NOT CONVINCED THAT FIBROMYALGIA CAN BE ELIMINATED NATURALLY? THEN READ:

- *The Fibromyalgia Relief Handbook*
  (Gives a full explanation of fibromyalgia—in plain English—and why so many people suffer from it, how to get relief from fibromyalgia symptoms, and more. This book is of vital importance to anyone suffering symptoms of fibromyalgia.)

36. NOT CONVINCED THAT THERE ARE NATURAL REMEDIES FOR VIRTUALLY EVERY DISEASE? THEN READ:

- *The Cure for All Diseases*
  (New research findings show that all diseases have simple explanations and cures once their true cause is known.)
- *Encyclopedia of Natural Medicine*
- *Health and Nutrition Secrets That Can Save Your Life*
  (Harness Your Body's Natural Healing Powers)
- *The Natural Physician's Healing Therapies: Proven Remedies That Medical Doctors Don't Know About*
- *Alternative Medicine: The Definitive Guide*
- *The Most Common Diseases & Their Alternative Natural Therapies*
- *The Most Effective Natural Medicines in the World*

37. NOT CONVINCED THAT YOU NEVER HAVE TO GET SICK? THEN READ:

- *You Can Be...Well At Any Age: Your Definitive Guide to Vibrant Health & Longevity*
  (For those seeking to ensure not only the maximum number of years to their lives, but the best possible quality to those years as well.)

- *How to Get Well—Handbook of Natural Healing*
  (Proven, effective solutions to your health problems—whatever they may be...An authoritative and practical manual on the most common ailments—and what you can do about them by a world-famous authority on nutrition and natural healing.)
- *Death by Diet*
- *The Food Revolution*
  (How Your Diet Can Help Save Your Life And Our World.)

38. NOT CONVINCED THAT PROPER DEEP BREATHING IS ONE OF THE MOST IMPORTANT AND BENEFICIAL THINGS YOU CAN DO? THEN READ:

- *Super Power Breathing for Super Energy, High Health & Longevity*
  (Live Longer, Healthier, Stronger With Every Breath! Empower Yourself—stimulate your body's natural healing & brain power; Energize Yourself—39 simple exercises for a vibrant, energized body; Relax Yourself—35 calming effects of a healthier, fitter body.)

39. NOT CONVINCED THAT YOUR LIVER ABSOLUTELY, POSITIVELY IS CLOGGED, CONGESTED, AND NEEDS CLEANSING, POTENTIALLY CURING A HOST OF ILLNESSES INCLUDING ALLERGIES, DIABETES, AND IRRITABLE BOWEL SYNDROME? THEN READ:

- *The Liver Cleansing Diet*
  (Love Your Liver And Live Longer.)
- *The Amazing Liver Cleanse*
  (A Powerful Approach To Improve Your Health and Vitality.)
- *The Healthy Liver & Bowel Book*
  (Detoxification Strategies for Your Liver & Bowel. Life Saving Strategies for those with many health problems, including liver disease, bowel problems and weight excess.)

40. NOT CONVINCED THAT THERE IS AN ALL-NATURAL CURE FOR DIABETES, AND THAT THE PHARMACEUTICAL INDUSTRY

OFFERED $30 MILLION TO TAKE IT OFF THE MARKET? THEN READ:

- *The Natural Diabetes Solution*

41. NOT CONVINCED THAT JUICING IS ABSOLUTELY NEEDED IF YOU WANT TO GET THE PROPER NUTRITION YOUR BODY NEEDS? THEN READ:
    - *The Juice Lady's Juicing For High-Level Wellness and Vibrant Good Looks*
    - *The Juice Lady™s Guide to Juicing for Health*
      (Unleashing the Healing Power of Whole Fruits and Vegetables. A Practical A-To-Z Guide to the Prevention and Treatment of the Most Common Health Disorders.
    - *The Ultimate Smoothie Book (Whip Up 101 Elixirs, Cordials, Tinctures and Teas to Boost Immunity and Enhance Well-Being.)*
    - *The Joy of Juicing*
      (Creative Cooking with Your Juicer. 150 imaginative, healthful juicing recipes for drinks, soups, salads, sauces, entrées, and desserts.)
    - *Power Juices Super Drinks*
      (Quick, Delicious Recipes to Prevent and Reverse Disease.)

42. NOT CONVINCED THAT JUICE FASTING IS THE MOST EFFECTIVE WAY TO LOSE WEIGHT, CLEANSE THE BODY OF IMPURITIES, INCREASE ENERGY, AND STIMULATE THE IMMUNE SYSTEM? THEN READ:
    - *Juice Fasting & Detoxification*
      (Use the Healing Power of Fresh Juice to Feel Young and Look Great. The fastest way to restore your health.)
    - *The Miracle of Fasting*
      (Proven Throughout History for Physical, Mental & Spiritual Rejuvenation.)

43. NOT CONVINCED THAT COLON CLEANSING IS ABSOLUTELY, POSITIVELY NEEDED BY EVERY SINGLE PERSON, AND THAT

DOING SO CAN ALLEVIATE ILLNESS AND DISEASE, INCREASE
METABOLISM AND POTENTIALLY SLOW OR REVERSE AGING?
THEN READ:

- *Cleanse & Purify Thyself "And I Will Exalt Thee to the Throne of Power"*
  (Highly effective intestinal cleansing; removes pounds of Disease-Causing Toxins and Disease-Causing Negative Emotions.)

- *The Detox Diet: The How to and When to Guide for Cleansing the Body of Chemicals, Toxins, Sugar, Caffeine, Nicotine, Alcohol, and More*

- *How to Cleanse and Detoxify Your Body Today!*
  (Finally…You Can Look And Feel Better! A body freer of toxins, mucus, acids, dead cells and all irritants is STRONGER, HEALTHIER & more VITAL.)

- *Internal Cleansing*
  (Rid Your Body of Toxins to Naturally and Effectively Fight: Heart Disease, Chronic Pain, Fatigue, PMS and Menopause Symptoms, Aging, Frequent Colds and Flu, Food Allergies.)

- *The Master Cleanser (with Special Needs and Problems)*

- *Healthy Living: A Holistic Guide to Cleansing, Revitalization and Nutrition*
  (Healthy Living: how fasting can save your life; how your body can rejuvenate itself, how you can achieve and maintain balanced health; how to improve your well-being; how you can prepare delicious vegetarian dishes including soups, entrées, salads, beverages and desserts. Features delicious all-natural vegetarian recipes.)

44. NOT CONVINCED THAT TOXINS LODGE IN THE FATTY TISSUE OF THE BODY AND ABSOLUTELY ARE CAUSING A HOST OF PHYSICAL AND MENTAL PROBLEMS AND MUST BE CLEANSED? THEN READ:

- *Clear Body, Clear Mind*
  (The Effective Purification Program.)

- *Purification: An Illustrated Answer to Drugs*

(Drugs cause the death of consciousness and awareness, and eventually of the body itself. If you value the ability to think clearly, emotional stability and a positive attitude about yourself, then *Purification: An Illustrated Answer to Drugs* is your answer.)

45. NOT CONVINCED THAT PROPER DIET CAN POTENTIALLY CURE ILLNESS AND LEAD TO VIBRANT HEALTH AND WELLNESS? THEN READ:

- *The 7 Steps to Perfect Health*
  (A practical guide to Mental, Physical, and Spiritual Wellness.)

- *The Ultimate Healing System*
  (The Illustrated Guide to Muscle Testing & Nutrition. A Breakthrough in Nutrition, Kinesiology, and Holistic Healing Techniques.)

- *Diet for a New America*
  (How Your Food Choices Affect Your Health, Happiness, and the Future of Life on Earth.)

- *Ultimate Lifetime Diet*
  (A Revolutionary All-Natural Program for Losing Weight and Building a Healthy Body.)

- *Getting Started on Getting Well*
  (A workbook and videos, which together provide adequate information for rebuilding the immune system so the body can then effectively fight the disease and heal itself as God designed.)

- *Official Know-It-All™ Guide to Health & Wellness*
  (Your Absolute, Quintessential, All You Wanted to Know, Complete Guide to wellness, disease prevention, and nutrition.)

- *Living Well: Taking Care of Your Health in the Middle and Later Years*
  (Easy-to-Use Decision Charts Quickly Show How to Treat Problems Yourself and When to See a Doctor.)

46. NOT CONVINCED THAT ENERGY EXISTS, AND ENERGY HEALING ABSOLUTELY WORKS? THEN READ:

- *The Healing Energy of Your Hands*
  (Demystifies the art of healing, beginning with a basic explanation of the nature of healing energy, illness and the role of the
  mind in the healing process. Offers techniques so simple that
  anyone, even a child, can work with healing energy.)

- *Quantum-Touch: The Power to Heal*
  (*Quantum-Touch* represents a major breakthrough in the art of
  hands-on healing. Whether you are a complete novice, a professional chiropractor, physical therapist, body worker, healer
  or other health professional, *Quantum-Touch* allows you a
  dimension of power in your work that heretofore had not
  seemed possible.)

- *Wheels of Light: Chakras, Auras, and the Healing Energy of the
  Body*
  (Explores the seven chakras, or energy centers, of the body
  with particular focus on the first charka, which has to do with
  our basic life force, our physical bodies and our sexuality.)

47. NOT CONVINCED THAT EATING MICROWAVED FOOD IS
    ABSOLUTELY DANGEROUS FOR YOUR HEALTH? THEN READ:

    - *Is Microwaved Food Killing Us?*

48. NOT CONVINCED THAT HYDROGENATED OIL AND TRANS
    FATS CAUSE HEART DISEASE AND A WHOLE HOST OF MED-
    ICAL PROBLEMS? THEN READ:

    - *Trans Fats: The Food Industry's Way of Giving You a Heart
      Attack*

49. NOT CONVINCED THAT EATING LOTS OF RAW ORGANIC
    FRUITS AND VEGETABLES CAN GIVE YOU DYNAMIC HEALTH?
    THE READ:

    - *Raw Foods: The Key to Eternal Youth*

50. NOT CONVINCED THAT MASS PRODUCED FOOD IS
    UNHEALTHY? THEN READ:

    - *Mass Produced Food: A Cancer in Every Box*

51. NOT CONVINCED THAT SUNSCREENS AND OTHER LOTIONS YOU PUT ON YOUR SKIN CAUSE CANCER AND OTHER DIS-EASES? THEN READ:

    - *What You Put on Your Skin is What Gives You Skin Cancer*

52. NOT CONVINCED THAT THE BODY NEEDS NATURAL SUNLIGHT AND THAT THE SUN DOES NOT CAUSE CANCER? THEN READ:

    - *Sunlight: The Missing Link to Health*

53. NOT CONVINCED THAT MAGNETIC FINGER AND TOE RINGS CAN REDUCE OR ELIMINATE PAIN, SLOW OR EVEN REVERSE THE AGING PROCESS, ALKALIZE THE BODY AND POTENTIAL-LY CURE MANY DISEASES? THEN READ:

    - *How to Reverse Aging and Eliminate Disease*

54. NOT CONVINCED THAT WATCHING TOO MUCH TELEVISION CAUSES THE BODY TO BECOME ACIDIC, LEADING TO DIS-EASE? THEN READ:

    - *Four Arguments for the Elimination of Television*

55. NOT CONVINCED THAT LACK OF SMILES, LOVE, HUGS, AND AFFECTION CAN CAUSE ILLNESS AND A HOST OF EMOTION-AL DISORDERS? THEN READ:

    - *The Medical Consequences of Loneliness*

56. NOT CONVINCED THAT YOUR WORDS, WHAT YOU SAY AND HOW YOU SAY IT, HAVE A POWERFUL IMPACT ON YOUR HEALTH AND SUCCESS? THEN READ:

    - *Should: How Habits of Language Shape Our Lives*
    - *What You Say Is What You Get*
    - *The Tongue: A Creative Force*

57. NOT CONVINCED THAT WRITING THINGS DOWN CAUSES THEM TO HAPPEN? THEN READ:

    - *Write it Down, Make it Happen*

58. NOT CONVINCED THAT THE SUPER RICH ARE GREEDY AND CORRUPT BEYOND BELIEF? THEN READ:

    - *Perfectly Rich*

59. NOT CONVINCED THAT YOU CAN EASILY LIVE TO BE OVER
100 YEARS OLD, NEVER GET SICK, AND THAT VIRTUALLY
EVERYTHING I'M SAYING IN THIS BOOK IS TRUE? THEN
READ:

- *How Long Do You Choose to Live? A Question of a Lifetime*
  (Imagine never needing another doctor again, having more athletic ability at seventy than you had at seventeen, perfect mental recall, and eternal youth. If the author can show you that
  these are more than wishful claims, that would interest you,
  wouldn't it? Read this book!)

- *Power Aging*

- *The 100 Simple Secrets of Healthy People*

- *Stopping the Clock*
  (Dramatic Breakthroughs in Anti-Aging and Age Reversal
  Techniques.)

- *The Longevity Strategy*
  (How to Live to 100 Using the Brain–Body Connection.)

- *Successful Aging*
  (Learn the surprising results of the MacArthur Foundation
  Study—the most extensive, comprehensive study on aging in
  America. Find out how the way you live—not the genes you
  were born with—determines health and vitality.)

- *The Okinawa Program*
  (How the World's Longest-Lived People Achieve Everlasting
  Health—And How You Can Too.)

- *On My Own at 107: Reflections on Life Without Bessie*
  (Sarah"Sadie" Delany's tribute to Bessie, her beloved younger
  sister and century-long companion who died...at age 104.)

- *Having Our Say: The Delany Sisters' First 100 Years*
  (The Delany Sisters on Family, Marriage, Taxes and Life...)

- *Living to 100*
  (Lessons in Living to Your Maximum Potential at Any Age.)

- *Centenarians: The Bonus Years*

(The book addresses the social and health needs of both the centenarian and their families or caretakers.)

- *If I Live to be 100*
  (Lessons from the Centenarians. This is a beautifully written and elegantly wise work that takes us inside the world of the very old and invites us to learn from them firsthand the art of living well for an exceptionally long period of time.)

- *On Being 100*
  (31 Centenarians Share Their Extraordinary Lives and Wisdom.)

- *Centenarians*
  (One Hundred 100-Year-Olds Who Made a Difference.)

All of these books are terrific. They give you more facts, more documentation and more inside information verifying and backing up everything I promote in this book. Please buy these books from us. The small profit we make will be used in our fight against healthcare fraud and corruption. If you have any questions about these books, or would like to buy them, go to www.naturalcures.com, or call 800-931-4721.

CHAPTER 12

The Cures for All Diseases

There are natural nondrug and nonsurgical cures for virtually every disease, illness and physical ailment. These cures are inexpensive and have virtually no negative side effects. I am not a doctor. I do not treat patients. According to the U.S. Government, I can not diagnose or treat disease. If I were to cure someone of cancer, I could go to jail for practicing medicine without a license. Therefore, I am presenting this information for educational purposes only.

I know that therapies such as energetic medicine, homeopathy, herbs, nutritional supplements and cleansing can help the body heal itself. What standard medicine attempts to do is to look at a person's symptoms, call it a "disease," and then prescribe drugs or surgery to suppress or eliminate the symptom. Unfortunately, medical doctors do not look for the cause, they only attempt to suppress the symptoms. If you simply suppress a symptom, you have not addressed the cause and the person will continue to get sick. Combine that with the new illnesses that are actually caused by the drugs themselves, and we find that a patient treated by a medical doctor with drugs and surgery continues to become sicker and sicker over time. A good example is a child who appears to have hyperactivity and a low attention span. He will probably be diagnosed with attention deficit disorder. Doctors will say that the child's brain chemistry is not right and needs a drug to fix the imbalance in the brain chemistry. The drug may have some short-term effects on balancing the brain chemistry, but the question that was missed is WHY the brain chemistry was unbalanced to begin with. What caused the chemical imbalance? If this was asked, we almost always find that food allergies, excitotoxins such as MSG and aspartame, and food additives are to blame. With simple dietary adjustments the brain chemistry becomes balanced and the child, in a matter of days, is no longer hyperactive and his attention span is back to normal.

Another example is when a person has pain, a doctor will give a drug to suppress the pain. All the drug does is stop the pain signals from reaching the brain. The cause of the pain is never addressed; if it is, we virtually always find the pain was caused by a blockage in electromagnetic impulses between cells. The Chinese actually discovered, over 2,000 years ago that with simple nondrug and nonsurgical procedures, the cause could be addressed and the pain eliminated permanently.

Imagine you are driving your car and the oil light goes on. That would be a symptom of a bigger problem. To "correct" the situation, you could simply take the bulb out. You stopped the symptom; the oil light is no longer illuminated. But you have not addressed the cause, continuing to run your car without oil, which will quickly cause major engine damage. The human body is the same way. Think about it this way, you don't have a headache because you have an aspirin deficiency.

The most important thing you can do is prevent disease and sickness. Most people wait until they have symptoms before seeking medical attention. In many cases the problem is so severe that major attention is needed. Imagine a person who never takes his car in for maintenance. One day the car starts making funny noises. The person does not immediately take the car in for service. He continues to drive the car, not realizing that the problem is getting worse and worse. The car finally stops running and must be towed in to the service station. The mechanic says all the bearings are worn out and must be replaced, a major engine overhaul. Our body is very similar. People run their bodies with aches and pains and symptoms, using drugs to suppress the symptoms without addressing the cause. One day the problem is so severe they seek medical attention and are told

"Your body is riddled with cancer," or "Your arteries are almost completely clogged and they need immediate bypass surgery." This would never happen if a person did basic maintenance of their body.

The pH test, in my opinion, is one of the simplest and best ways to determine your health potential. If your saliva and urine pH is alkaline, disease and sickness virtually can not exist. Remember, most serious medical conditions such as cancer, heart disease, arthritis and any pain in general did not develop overnight. The condition was developing for years before you ever noticed a symptom. I was asked one time what I would do if I found out I had cancer or heart disease. My response was that that was virtually impossible since I routinely check my body pH and monitor my arteries. Blocked arteries, for example, develop over years. I would know if my arteries were beginning to clog years before any major blockages. If I discovered this, I would utilize natural treatments such as nutritional therapy, and chelation. I would then review my condition to see if it stayed the same, got worse or got better. The key element is that I would know years in advance of any major problem.

The good news is that even if you do have a major problem, there are natural alternatives to drugs and surgery in most cases. I realize that what I present in this book is said to be unconventional. However, throughout history "conventional" has always been what the majority believed to be true. Those who were in the minority were classified as heretics. The conventional wisdom at one time was that the sun revolved around the earth. Anyone who thought that the earth revolved around the sun was a fool and a heretic. At one time the conventional wisdom was the earth was obviously flat, and anyone who suggested the earth was round was a fool and a heretic. At one time the conventional wisdom was man will never build a machine that can fly, anyone who thought otherwise was a fool and a heretic. As early as the 1970s, the conventional wisdom within the scientific community was food and nutrition had absolutely nothing to do with health, disease, or illness. Anyone who suggested good nutrition could play a major role in preventing and curing disease was a heretic.

I would like to give you the cures for virtually every disease; I would like to tell you the natural treatments available that can eliminate your symptoms and, at the same time, address the cause instead of simply suppressing the symptom. However, as I began to write this book the Federal Trade Commission and the Food and Drug Administration took unprecedented action. I am forbidden to give you specific cures in this book. The FTC has ordered me NOT to give you any specific product recommendations, or say where you can acquire the cures and receive treatment. And you thought we had free speech in America. You thought that the First Amendment of the U.S. Constitution protected our rights to speak our opinions freely. This simply is not true. We do not have free speech in America when it comes to healthcare. I can write a book about how to build a nuclear bomb. I can write a book on how to be a terrorist. I can write a book filled with pornographic images. I can write a book accusing politicians and big business of corruption. I can write a book filled with bigotry, hate and prejudice. I can write a book about my alien abduction. I can write a book about how I talk to the dead and see angels. All of this is protected by free speech. But I can not write a book and tell you how to cure your cancer without chemotherapy and surgery.

This entire chapter has been censored by the FTC. If you are as outraged as I am, you will join me in fighting this censorship. Just imagine for a moment what is happening here. I am not allowed to tell you my opinions in this book. How many millions of people will needlessly suffer and die because they are not allowed to know the truth about effective, inexpensive natural cures? However, there is a way you can get this information. If you go to www.naturalcures.com and become a private member, you will have access to all of this data. You can even e-mail me any question, and either I or my staff will give you the answers you seek. It is important for you to know that the very first step that you must take if you want to be healthy, prevent, or cure any disease is to take personal responsibility. Do not rely on the pharmaceutical industry, the scientists and researchers, the medical doctors, your insurance company, government agencies, or politicians; you must take charge and take full responsibility for your health.

A week ago I met a woman who recognized me from television. Her son was diagnosed with attention deficit disorder. He was incredibly hyperactive, and his attention span was almost nil. He failed every exam in school and was disruptive to the class. She wondered if she should take the doctor's advice and give the child Ritalin. I suggested that she see some healthcare practitioners who use all-natural treatments instead of drugs and surgery. I asked what the child ate, trying to get her to be as specific as possible. I said simply eliminate all dairy products, white sugar, white flour, aspartame, and MSG. I wrote down for her recommended meals and educated her on how to read food labels. She became very encouraged and excited about the possibility, yet remained skeptical that such a simple change could make such a profound difference. I gave her my number asked her to call me, as I was curious to know the results. Three days later she called. This woman was out of her mind. She told me that she absolutely could not believe the change in her child. The hyperactivity was virtually gone and the child's attention span and ability to concentrate was near 100 percent. For the first time in two years the child sat at the dinner table and ate his meal like a normal, well-mannered person. She even received a phone call from the child's teacher, who could not believe the change that had happened.

These kinds of stories happen all the time. Whether your concern is cancer, heart disease, arthritis, heartburn, PMS, headaches, pain, insomnia, acne, lupus, asthma, herpes, sexual dysfunction, yeast infections, ADD, snoring, diabetes, depression, anxiety, stress, etc., there is a simple, effective natural solution. I am sorry that I can not list all the remedies in this book. The FTC and FDA have promised to prosecute me if I tell you the products to use that cure or prevent disease.

Keep in mind that I am not compensated in any way from any of the products that I recommend. I have no conflicts of interest. I only make money when you purchase the books and other informational material that I sell. I use much of this money to educate the public and continue with my research. I also use this money to fight against corruption in the pharmaceutical industry and government. Please know that you can prevent and virtually cure almost every disease without drugs and surgery. Please know that you can live a life full of energy and vitality, and virtually never get sick.

CHAPTER 13

The Solution

Over the years there have been a few individuals, such as Ralph Nader, who have done a commendable job of exposing corruption in government and big business. There have been a few pure consumer advocate groups that have been untainted by the lure and influence of big business money and government pressure. These individuals and groups have educated Americans and the world through the use of books, public appearances, newsletters, and recently, internet web sites. Although they have done a commendable job two major problems still exist.

1. Even with this information out in the public, the mainstream media has still suppressed and watered down their message. In surveys, 80 percent of Americans are still totally unaware of the massive corporate and government corruption that adversely affects their way of life.

2. These organizations and individuals only expose the fraud, deceptions, and corruptions that exist. They do little to actually cause things to change; therefore, very little has changed and, in fact, things are worse now than ever before.

I believe that the only way to effect change is as follows.

1. The majority of people must be made aware of corporate and governmental corruption. The majority must be exposed to the truth of how "it's all about the money," at the expense of the average person.

253

Therefore, my mission is to not only write the books, newsletters, and websites exposing the truth, but also to invest my fortune in promoting these books, newsletters and websites throughout the television, radio and print media. The challenge is already evident. The Federal Trade Commission has already taken action denying me my First Amendment right of free speech by forbidding me to publish my opinions in book form and marketing them. The mainstream media is also suppressing my ability to run advertising promoting these books, newsletters and websites. However, it must be done. The information must get out to as many people as possible as soon as possible if change is ever going to occur. The corrupt corporations, corporate executives, politicians and government agencies must be exposed.

2. In addition to educating the public on how they are being deceived by big corporations and the government, if change is to occur aggressive action must be taken against the corporations, government agencies, and individual corporate executives and politicians. In addition to educating the public, it is my intention to spearhead lawsuits—specifically, class action lawsuits—against those who are allowing millions of people to suffer needlessly through suppression of the truth about natural nondrug and nonsurgical cures. Since class action suits have been filed against the tobacco industry, things have slowly begun to change in that area. The same will happen in healthcare. As of right now, no one is taking the lead in fighting the pharmaceutical industry. Together we can create a society where fewer people get sick with disease and illness, instead of the current trend where more people every year become sick with disease and illness.

Doesn't it make you mad knowing that corporate executives are knowingly and purposely putting chemicals in our food that make you fat and give you disease? Wouldn't you like those big greedy corporations to pay for their actions? I would.

In order to do this, my newly-launched website, www.natural cures.com, will be at the forefront of educating people and finding people who want to join in and reap the financial benefits of class action lawsuits against the big corporations that have been deceiving us for decades. When you go to www.naturalcures.com you must become a private member. This allows me to exercise my First Amendment right of free speech. The benefits of being a private member are:

- Subscription to the monthly newsletter *Natural Cures*. Each month I and my staff will read dozens of natural healthcare newsletters and reports. Since many of these reports and newsletters are owned by companies that sell various supplements and products, there is a potential conflict of interest and their advice could be swayed by the profit motive of getting you to buy the supplements they sell. Since we accept no advertising and do not sell supplements, we are unbiased. My *Natural Cures* newsletter will give you up-to-the-minute new breakthrough discoveries in alternative natural health. We will summarize for you all of the information that is being published so that you can learn this information in a fraction of the time it would take you to read and understand all of the newsletters independently.

- Each month my staff and I will be reading the most current natural healing books on the market and provide you with short summaries of all the newest information.

- Each month we will tell you the newest breakthroughs in natural cures.

- On the *Natural Cures* website I will list dozens of books by many different authors on various subjects relating to everything I've touched on in this book. It is important to know that there are dozens of authors who have published books that contain life saving information; unfortunately, these books are suppressed and never get out to the public. I will use this website to promote the authors and their books, allowing you access to information that has virtually never been available before. It will be like opening Pandora's box and exposing you to the secrets of healthcare that have been hidden behind closed doors for decades.

- The website will list practically every disease or ailment known, and give you the specific natural remedies for curing and preventing those diseases.

- The website will tell you what "all-natural" vitamins, minerals, herbs, and supplements you should AVOID. Greed shows no boundaries. There are people in the vitamin and food supplement business who are only in it for the money. You need to know what products to stay away from, as well as specific products that actually work. This section alone is invaluable. You may be spending hundreds of dollars on worthless food supplements and not know it.

- The website will allow you to e-mail me directly with any question you have. I or my staff will give you a prompt response. We will also list the most commonly asked questions and their answers. This is one of the most valuable benefits of this website. I meet people all over the world who are sick, or have pain or some sort of medical condition. The number one complaint I have is that people do not know where to get information that they can trust about natural alternative therapies. They don't know who to ask, what to believe or what to do. So they go to their medical doctor and do whatever they're told because they don't know what else to do. Now you have a place where you can ask any question regarding natural alternative preventative measures and cures. Not only can we give you answers, but we can also give you specialized books, websites, and healthcare practitioners so that you can prevent and cure your medical condition without drugs and surgery.

- The website will also allow you to express how you have been misled, deceived, and lied to by the big corporations and/or government agencies. Your horror stories may be listed on the website if you permit us. This will allow you to read what others have experienced, and also allow others to read your experience. This also allows you to join in class action lawsuits from which, if they result in monetary damages being paid, you could receive your fair share.

Individually we are powerless against the big corporations and the government agencies that run unpoliced. Together as a group we can be a powerful force that will change healthcare for the better. As a group we can demand that the food we buy in supermarkets and restaurants be free of chemicals and food additives. We can demand that we have free access and freedom of choice regarding natural alternative treatments and therapies. As a group we can demand that the advertising we are exposed to no longer be deceitful, misleading and fraudulent. As a group we can create a society where there is less sickness and disease, where we live longer with more energy and vitality than ever before, and where we eat delicious foods and are not condemned to being fat. Please go to www.naturalcures.com and become a member. The information you will have access to can change your life for the better in so many ways it will be hard to imagine. If you do not have access to the internet, my monthly newsletter *Natural Cures* can be mailed to you. Call 800-931-4721 for more information.

I am determined to change healthcare in America and the world. I am picking up where Ralph Nader left off. I am a true, pure consumer advocate. My motto is "empowering the powerless." Please join me.

CHAPTER 14

A True FDA Horror Story

On my website, www.naturalcures.com, there will be hundreds of true, real life horror stories of how the FDA and FTC persecute individuals, and how these government agencies protect the profits of big business. Rarely, if ever, are these abuses of power exposed. Most people do not realize that these agencies act as judge, jury and executioner. The individuals and small businesses that they attack are virtually power-less against these out-of-control, ruthless agencies. When you read these stories you will begin to feel like the Gestapo is operating in America. Remember, when the citizens of this country stand up and make their collective voices heard, change will occur. Here is one such story as told firsthand by the victim himself, as outlined in an open let-ter to President Carter. This is reprinted with permission.

An Open Letter to President Carter
Subject: Unjust & Unwarranted Bureaucratic Harassment That Will Result In The Loss of A Large Number of Jobs In Ohio

I have a most urgent and serious matter. I called your office but got your secretary. She told me I could not talk to you and also that you do not return calls. She said the only way to get in touch with you was write a letter. I could not do this, for a letter would take too long to both reach you and have you return it. This is a matter that needs attention immediately.

In your main campaign promise, you said that you would reform the bureaucracy to a point where it was responsive and helpful to the American people. At this point, myself and many other people associated with me here in Ohio would like to take you up on your promise.

I am writing to report gross irregularities by one federal agency that is under your administration. This agency is about to unjustly jeopardize the jobs and livelihood of presently over 250 people here in Ohio and other states, and in the near future, thousands of people. Also, actions by this agency indicate the possible existence of irregularities of scandalous proportions.

Ohio has already been hard hit by the loss of 5,000 jobs in the steel industry, which a new government report indicates was a direct result of over-regulation by the bureaucracy.

With regard to our problem, until you have had a chance to review the matter, I will not name the agency or the product which will tip off which agency it is.

I am not a crusader, and although I vote, I have little interest in politics. I am a small businessman. I started my business ten years ago with my own money and initiative. I was nearly flat broke when I started, was working for a large corporation and I had to struggle for the first five years to become successful. I am what you might call proof that the American system works, and what America is all about, the very basis for the start of this country – that any man who chooses to go into any enterprise he wishes and through as much hard work as he is willing to put into it make a profit and pursue life, liberty and happiness. Now that did happen. In the past five years, although my business has been small, it has been very successful. And things were going well—up until now.

About three years ago, my wife and I developed a new product, initially by accident, that helped relieve an unpleasant and unwanted condition faced by a large percentage of the population. We didn't think of it as a commercial product then, but used it faithfully ourselves. As we let friends try it, more and more of them raved about it and wanted the product also. Everybody told us we should market the product. However, we were reluctant because it was a product line which was completely different from the product line in which we were then engaged.

About six months ago we made the decision to go ahead and market the product. My wife and I had consistently used it for three years to this point, and I was really sold on its merit because not only did it have a good initial effect, but the effect was long-term, and seemingly indefinite. I then tested the product on several hundred people with resounding success. This was the law imperious I needed to implement the marketing of this product.

The product is legitimate and valid. There are similar products like it on the market but much less effective, in our opinion. You can see if it works in a few minutes. You don't need complicated tests by a team of "experts"; I am willing to send this express mail—which only takes twenty-four hours—any number of these products that you want to test yourself or to test by your staff.

Initial sales and customer response indicate that this will be one of the fastest growing products of recent times. This product in a few short years will create a new industry employing thou-

sands of people. The product is already responsible for the creation of hundreds of jobs here in Ohio and many more from out-of-state suppliers.

Now for the bad news. We were told by many business colleagues prior to marketing this product that this product competes with many large, established businesses and organizations who have powerful lobbies. We were told that these established companies and organizations had an "in" with one government agency, and through this agency they would stop the product. We laughed it off at the time as an old wives' tale. We had never had any trouble before, but it was true that all our previous products did not compete with any large businesses or organizations.

In the past two months of marketing and producing this product, the following incredible events occurred in the following chronological order:

1. In the initial state of implementing this product we went to the agency in question here. We asked them for a list of rules and regulations we had to comply with to market and produce this product. We were

told that no such list of rules and regulations existed and that it was simply a common sense judgment of an agency investigator. We tried three different offices of this agency to come up with these regulations, but were unsuccessful. There also seems to be no experts on this agency, professionals, consultants, etc.

2. We drew up a set of standards for our product that we would have drawn up anyway which we felt would be even much stronger and higher than any of those of the agency. We tested the product, we had lab tests on our product, the product was closely quality controlled, and we were told by the laboratory people and suppliers in the product line that they knew of no other company with such high standards and who took so much care in the production of their product. In fact, our lab reports showed a quality ten times greater than the best known brands of existing similar products.

3. Upon seeking suppliers for various productions steps of our product, we were appalled at the gross negligence regarding consumer safety of the majority of these suppliers. All of these suppliers that we felt were grossly negligent had, in fact, been inspected and approved by the agency in question. In fact, many of these inspections were very recent.

On the eve of the production of the product, the agency sent inspectors to compile information on our product. Again, we asked them for help—a list of rules and regulations that we had to comply with. Again, they said they knew nothing of such rules and that it was a common sense judgment. We asked them other pointed questions about the production of the product. We found these agents to be totally ignorant and can not understand how they can even be working at the job.

Now, after starting the entire process and spending all the money for marketing and all the money for supplies, when we actually started production, then the inspectors from this agency came in with a very long, detailed, documented list of regulations and rules—*the same list we requested and they said did not exist.* Even though we had taken all the precautions, they cited us for "violations of 29 rules." We were in violation of a few of the 29 alleged rules; however, these were items we were ignorant about and were items that would not be thought of even with common sense judgment. However, a majority of the alleged violations were petty nonsense and exaggerated stretchings of interpretations. However, the point that hit us the hardest is that all 29 alleged violations were present in nearly every other supplying establishment that we had been in and that had, in fact, been approved by this same agency, it became obvious at this point that we were being subjected to a double standard and outright harassment.

4. Irate, I called the chief administrator of the regional office of the agency. I called him to complain about the following:
   a. Why wasn't I given a list of rules and regulations to comply with when I asked for them prior to my starting the production?
   b. Why did he initially send in such ignorant and inexperienced people to us first?
   c. How could it be possible that I had chosen the highest quality supplier that I had found in Ohio and that he would be guilty of so many rule infringements when most of the other establishments were so grossly negligent and still passed this inspection?
   d. As a taxpayer, I wanted to know why this agency was so lax to begin with to allow such negligence to exist.

The administrator became arrogant at this point and claimed he knew of no such double standards, etc., and that not only were we going to have trouble with the production of this product, but that he was reclassifying it as another product in which he had the power to debate legally within the realm of his agency. His reclassification of the product was so ludicrous that it defied belief that anybody could come up with this reclassification using the farthest stretch of the imagination. He then told me that the product was mislabeled as to claims. I asked him if he or his agency had tried or tested the product. He said no and that he did not intend to. At that point I blew up and said, "How in the world could anyone say a product does not meet label claims if they have not even tried or tested the product?" At this point he told us that "we should get out of this line of business and, if we didn't, he was going to make big trouble for us." I couldn't believe this gangland style threat coming from my own government. I told him at that point that I had a legitimate, valid, high-quality product and that I was going to defend it to the hilt and that contrary to what he may be thinking I was not going to buckle under to this unjust tyranny and bullying tactics.

If what is going on with this agency is not an isolated incident and is being carried out for the reasons that we highly suspect at this point, the implications are ominous. It means conspiracy by a government agency to engage in antitrust actions. It means that free enterprise does not exist and that the major freedom that this country stands for has been striped away from the common man. This situation in the future will create hardship and crisis for everyone concerned, including those benefiting from the present monopolies, for their benefits will be short lived. Humans as animals do not become vicious until they are trapped.

This situation also has serious detrimental effects on the economy. The more entrepreneurs you stop, the less jobs, the less quality of existing goods will occur resulting in a lower standard of living. It means no free market.

Now we are presently investigating this matter ourselves and are filing a complaint with the anti-trust division of the justice department. However, it is critical that we get immediate help. The only person who can supply this help is you. Here's why: I don't know how such a situation occurred, that this agency has the power of judge, jury, and executioner. They can literally sit there and play God. Their attitude is horrendous. Somehow they have lost sight of the fact that they are public servants and are there to provide for the welfare of the

American people. Instead of helping and expediting a business in carrying out regulations, they do everything in their power to disrupt and stop enterprise with total disregard for impact on both the business and public. Somehow, this agency has construed that the American taxpayer is there to serve them. With the powers to delay production of a product without a trial, they will, in fact, produce the same results as if they had prosecuted and won, because by stopping a product by two years, you put the company out of business and you allow competitors to step in and reap the fruits of this company's labor.

There is a little bit of good news out of all of this. This is my first negative encounter with a government agency. I have dealt with many government agencies in the past, and contrary to popular belief, have found them competent, helpful and honest. It appears the job of revamping the bureaucracy may be big, but not impossible, for it seems that the problems are isolated to certain agencies.

Knowing the situation, would you please get back to us as soon as possible? Please contact me, Benjamin Suarez, President, P.C.A., 4626 Cleveland Avenue N., Canton, Ohio 44767, (216) 494-5065.

In fairness to all concerned, we will print the net result of our inquiry to you, step by step as the events transpire right here in this same paper. As the owner of the business (the burden all owners bear) I will take the liability for the above letter. However, the following is a plea from workers who stand the loss of employment if the actions of the described agency are left unchallenged.

If you would like more information on Mr. Suarez's product, go to www.naturalcures.com and become a private member.

Glossary

Acupressure

A massage technique which stimulates pressure points on the surface of the body to promote circulation, derived from ancient Chinese methods. See also *Therapeutic Massage*.

Acupuncture

A technique of Asian medicine, performed only by licensed healthcare providers, in which fine needles are inserted into the body at specific points to promote circulation. It typically involves insertion of needles, but includes the techniques of electro-acupuncture, cupping or moxibustion. For more information, visit Acupuncture.com.

Alexander Technique®

A somatic education method that develops and maintains the alignment of the head, neck and back in order to reduce unnecessary strains on the body, and improve posture and overall health.

Biofeedback

A training technique to consciously regulate normal body functions such as heart rate, breathing, brain activity levels and body temperature. This technique helps to change physical responses to stress as well as enhance overall health. Training is guided by both a trained practitioner and simple electronic devices that monitor body functions and provide feedback.

CranioSacral Therapy

A manual therapy that involves a gentle, non-invasive palpation (touch by the practitioner) of the head, spinal column, and sacrum.

Cupping

An Asian medical technique which utilizes a glass or bamboo cup to create suction on the skin above a painful muscle or acupuncture point.

Electro-acupuncture

An Asian medical technique which uses mild, low-voltage electric stimulation of acupuncture points.

Feldenkrais Method®
A somatic education method taught in an individual or group setting that uses verbal and hands-on guidance to improve posture and flexibility. For more information, visit Feldenkrais Guild of North America at www.feldenkraisguild.com. See also *Hanna Somatics.*

Guided Imagery
Interactive Guided Imagery ℠ is a process using the power of the mind to evoke a positive physical response. Guided Imagery can reduce stress and slow the heart rate, stimulate the immune system and reduce pain. For more information, visit The Guided Imagery Resource Center online.

Hanna Somatics®
A somatic education method derived from Feldenkrais that uses slow-motion movement techniques to release unconscious and habitual muscle tensions.

Herbal Medicine
An Asian medical practice for the prescription of therapeutic foods or herbs.

Manual Lymph Drainage
A massage technique which uses gentle, rhythmic pressure to stimulate lymphatic flow.

Manual Therapies
Any hands-on technique, especially therapeutic manipulation of body structure, e.g., deep tissue or connective tissue. See also *CranioSacral Therapy, Myofascial Release, Polarity Therapy, Reflexology, Reiki, Rolfing®, Rosen Method®, Therapeutic Touch®* and *Trigger Point /Myotherapy.*

Massage
Any hands-on technique for relaxation or health enhancement. For more information, visit American Massage Therapy Association. See also *Shiatsu Massage, Sports Massage, Swedish Massage* and *Therapeutic Massage.*

Moxibustion

An Asian medical technique for the application of heat to an acupuncture point by burning an herb called moxa (artemisia vulgaris) near the skin or on top of a slice of ginger.

Myotherapy

See *Trigger Point/Myotherapy*.

Myofascial Release

A manual therapy technique which works on underlying connective tissue or trigger points to facilitate the release of chronic muscular tensions restricting posture, movement and circulation.

Nutrition Counseling

Qualified practitioners provide nutritional counseling and education through one-on-one sessions as well as group classes. A variety of topics are covered, including weight management, nutrition for health and wellness, and vegetarian eating. Practitioners in this field include both licensed dietitians and nutrition counselors. For more information, visit the American Dietetic Association at www.eatright.org or Nutrition Navigator at http://navigator.tufts.edu.

Polarity Therapy

A manual therapy that combines the holding of pressure points and gentle stretching to balance the body's energy.

Qi Gong

An ancient "soft" Chinese martial art form combining movement, mindful meditation and focused breathing as a means of cultivating qi, or chi, throughout the body for perceived health benefits and spiritual insights. The slow gentle movements are thought to promote self-healing, strengthen the immune system, release tension and stimulate vitality. Tai Chi, which has more complex movements, originated from the practice of Qi Gong.

Reflexology

A manual therapy which uses pressure applied to reflex zones on the feet corresponding to other body areas. See also *Therapeutic Massage*.

Reiki
A manual therapy in which the practitioner's palms are held over the body to direct the flow of life energy in the manner of a laying-on of hands technique.

Rolfing® (Structural Integration)
A manual therapy which manipulates deep tissue to bring the major segments of the body-head, shoulder, thorax, pelvis and legs-into a better vertical alignment with gravity. For more information, visit The Rolf Institute at www.rolf.org.

Rosen Method®
A manual therapy which uses gentle touch and verbal exchange between practitioner and client to help draw the client's attention to areas of tension.

Shiatsu
A massage technique which applies pressure to points and meridians on the surface of the body.

Somatic Education
Any body education method for improved balance, posture, integration and/or ease of movement. The two most common methods are the Alexander Technique® and the Feldenkrais Method®. See also *Hanna Somatics®*.

Sports Massage
Any techniques used to assist an athlete to train or perform, but especially Swedish massage or joint movement, relaxation and mobilization techniques.

Swedish Massage
This most common form of massage uses strokes, manipulations and movements to stimulate, relax or rehabilitate the body.

Tai Chi ("Tai chi chuan")
An ancient "soft" Chinese martial art form and a means of cultivating the qi, or chi, for perceived health benefits and spiritual insights. Tai

chi originally stemmed from the ancient practice of qi gong, and consists of many qi gong movements, but has evolved to a distinct and separate martial art form. The slow gentle movements are thought to promote strength, balance, health, vitality, and an over-all sense of well-being.

Therapeutic Massage
Any massage for health enhancement (for example, acupressure, Swedish, neuromuscular or reflexology) as opposed to massage strictly for pleasure or relaxation.

Therapeutic Touch®
A manual therapy akin to laying-on of hands, in which the practitioner's palms are held near the body to affect the energetic fields.

Trigger Point/Myotherapy
A manual therapy technique which releases knots of muscle tension which refer pain to other areas, followed by gentle stretches or movement to retrain the muscles.

Yoga
An ancient practice that strengthens and tones muscle and improves balance and flexibility, while increasing blood flow and vitality. While there are six distinct forms of yoga, most involve physical movements and holding of postures, while incorporating breathing and mindful attention. Many of the yoga studios incorporate a blend of yoga styles and offer a variety in levels of rigor.

About the Author

Kevin Trudeau is fast becoming the nation's foremost consumer advocate. Knowing from firsthand experience the power of greed, Kevin pled guilty to felonies in his youth and spent almost two years in prison realizing that "the love of money" is the root of all evil. Kevin then reprioritized his life. His new business and personal mission statement became "We positively impact the whole person." Since then, Kevin has been involved in a vast array of business enterprises that marketed or sold products that Kevin personally used and believed in 100 percent. He is personally responsible for over $2 billion in business worldwide. Having been attacked and sued in three continents, Kevin knows from personal experience how big business and government try to debunk individuals who promote products that could hurt the profits of the giant multinational corporations. Today Kevin spends most of his time spearheading www.naturalcures.com, the website that promotes education about natural healing therapies; and the www.thewhistleblower.com, the website that exposes corporate and government abuse and corruption. Kevin is actively pursuing lawsuits against the individuals, corporations and government agencies that take advantage of the average consumer. He is also dedicated to the formation of various foundations to pursue these goals, and has donated much of his fortune for that purpose. Kevin is available for personal appearances, seminars, and book signings on a limited basis. Call 800-931-4721 for more information. If outside the U.S.A., please call +1 847-850-1476 for any information, to order any books, or subscriptions to the Natural Cures Newsletter.